in General Practice

Pocket Examiner
in

# General Practice

Anthony Reed

MBBS, FRCGP, DRCOG

*General Practitioner*
*Penrith, Cumbria*

PITMAN

PITMAN PUBLISHING LIMITED
128 Long Acre, London WC2E 9AN

*Associated Companies*
Pitman Publishing Pty Ltd, Melbourne
Pitman Publishing New Zealand Ltd, Wellington

Distributed in the United States of
America and Canada by Urban &
Schwarzenberg Inc., 7 East Redwood
Street, Baltimore, MD 21202

First Published 1984


British Library Cataloguing in Publication Data

Reed, Anthony
    Pocket examiner in general practice.
    1. Family medicine—Problems, exercises, etc.
    I. Title
    610'.76        RC58

ISBN 0 272 79738 3

© Anthony Reed, 1984

Text set in 9/10pt Palatino Roman
Printed and bound in Great Britain at The Pitman Press, Bath

# Contents

# Introduction

It is the intention of any examination to test the examinee's knowledge of the course curriculum. In a subject as broadly based as general practice it is understandable that this curriculum will be extensive. Ability in any subject can be broken down into terms of:

1 Knowledge
2 Skills
3 Attitudes

This holds good for general practice. At undergraduate level you will not be expected to have the expertise of a mature general practitioner but you have seen primary care operate and observed its strengths and weaknesses.

Let us examine 1, 2 and 3 in greater detail

1 The knowledge base includes not only a working expertise in hospital specialities but also a detailed knowledge of general practice areas, e.g. acute paediatric infections, the early signs of illness, diseases rarely referred out of primary care, patterns of chronic illness etc.

   In addition there are non-clinical areas such as human behaviour and development, practice administration and the structure of the NHS.
2 Skills include not only the practical examples of physical examination but the ability to interpret human behaviour, both verbal and non-verbal.
3 Attitude is perhaps the most difficult area to evaluate. Students must appreciate, however, that in general practice it is people who present with problems and not interesting clinical syndromes carried by a host.

The very heart of general practice is the consultation. This is the situation when a patient confides in his/her doctor. Here the primary care physician analyses the problem in terms of the physical, social and psychological aspects. The relevance of each of these areas in every case is evaluated before the patient's problem can be defined. Once the problem has been clarified then possible solutions for the patient can be generated. Each solution must take account of the physical, psychological and social

1

aspects for that particular patient. Here, knowledge of the patient and his/her background is of paramount importance. The general practitioner has this unique knowledge and, therefore, solutions are likely to be more acceptable to the patient.

Consider a fairly common problem presented by mothers: that of insomnia in a toddler. We are well aware that this is almost always a behavioural problem and that it is an interaction of maternal anxiety and an attention seeking measure in the baby. Some mothers merely require this to be pointed out. Others consider themselves to be failures because they require medical advice. Occasionally a mother cannot accept that the baby is completely well. In certain situations it is acceptable to suggest that the child may merely require to be left alone after checking that there is no obvious physical cause. In certain households it is not possible to leave the baby to cry because other children may be disturbed or even because the parents are sharing the child's bedroom.

You will see, therefore, that you must be sensitive to the patient's situation and often the 'textbook' answer is not appropriate.

The remainder of this book is designed to give you a foretaste of the examination and to help you prepare properly for something which is not an ordeal but rather a true test of a 'balanced' practitioner.

I doubt if I can coach a poor candidate to enable him to pass, but I hope I can encourage a timid student that by correct preparation he will give a more realistic representation of his actual ability. Too often a candidate thinks that by saying little he is not making mistakes. This may be true, but neither is he gaining marks or impressing his examiner with his personality or sensitivity. The worth of a good practitioner is in part measured by this 'presentability' to patients, for an uncommunicative doctor will not be able to obtain a good history and, therefore, will be less likely to define a problem. Your examiner is well aware of this facility and your ability to generate possible solutions to a problem can be compared to your ability to help patients with their problems.

Naturally this book is not a definitive test, but merely a vehicle to stimulate your wider reading. A comprehensive reading list is included.

# 2
# Questions

## CLINICAL MEDICINE

### A Infective and parasitic diseases

1 In a child with gastroenteritis what is the most important clinical feature which must be assessed?

2 Describe the presentation and treatment of scarlet fever.

3 What are the presenting features of measles?

4 What are Koplik's spots?

5 What are the principles of management of whooping cough?

6 Can a patient with chickenpox cause a contact to develop shingles?

7 What is the major drug to avoid in suspected infectious mononucleosis?

8 What clinical pointers make you suspect Legionnaire's disease?

9 What is the major problem in treating patients with tuberculosis?

10 What is the purpose of having a notifiable disease register?

11 When a traveller from abroad presents with a fever what are the important management points?

12 What are the important factors in the collection and transmission of urine samples?

13 What is the mechanism of fever production in febrile illness?

3

14 What are the reasons for NOT prescribing antibiotics in cases of undiagnosed fever?

15 What are the requirements for an effective general practice immunization programme?

16 What are the features of toxocariasis in children?

17 How best can toxocariasis be prevented from infecting humans?

18 What are the commonest causes of 'worms' in children and what are the mainstays of treatment?

## B Endocrine disorders and disorders of metabolism

19 What are the major objectives for the management of diabetes?

20 What are the three types of diabetic syndrome?

21 What is the place of oral hypoglycaemic agents in the treatment of diabetes?

22 Why do late onset diabetics fail to adhere to their recommended diets?

23 Why might a previously stable diabetic become hypoglycaemic when treated for angina?

24 What are the psychosocial problems which need to be discussed with adolescent diabetics?

25 What are the endocrinological causes of weight loss of recent onset?

26 How is it possible to tell clinically between a thyrotoxic patient and one with an anxiety state?

27 What is the management of a patient with thyrotoxicosis who develops a sore throat while on treatment?

28 Are there any circumstances when slow intro-

duction of thyroid hormone is indicated in the treatment of myxoedema?

29 What is the commonest presentation of thyrotoxicosis in the elderly?

30 Most obese patients believe it is their 'glands' to blame. What are the rare organic causes of obesity?

31 What is the management of obesity in general practice?

32 When is amenorrhoea physiological?

33 What is the timing of pubertal features in normal males?

34 How does osteoporosis present to the general practitioner?

35 In the management of infertility, what is of paramount importance?

36 How should you manage the treatment of alcoholism in general practice?

37 Why should a child who has had a moderate or large amount of alcohol be observed in hospital?

38 Cushing's disease can be mimicked by a more common problem in general practice. What is it?

39 In anorexia nervosa what are the factors that influence prognosis?

## C  Diseases of blood and blood-forming organs

40 What is a normal ESR?

41 What are the physical signs of anaemia?

42 How common is glossitis in iron deficiency anaemia?

43 What are the principles of management of iron deficiency?

44 What is the best form of oral medication for iron deficiency anaemia?

45 Why might a patient request parenteral iron therapy instead of tablets and what major argument may you use to dissuade him?

46 In iron deficiency anaemia what are the causes of failure to respond to oral iron therapy?

47 You are contacted by a young mother ringing from home who has a child who has just swallowed a bottle full of her iron tablets. What do you do?

48 In rheumatoid arthritis what is the commonest form of anaemia?

49 Name three conditions which can occur in a treated case of pernicious anaemia.

50 It is common for patients on B12 injections to come every 3 weeks demanding their 'top-up' and to say they know it was due because they were feeling tired.

51 What is the likely diagnosis in a patient with a macrocytosis and a normal haemoglobin level?

52 In the elderly, what is the commonest cause of idiopathic thrombocytopenic purpura (ITP)?

53 What are the features you would look for if a mother asked if her child has leukaemia?

54 In children with acute leukaemia are there any contraindications to immunization routines?

55 What are the principles of clinical management of a patient with chronic lymphatic leukaemia (CLL)?

56 Is there any way in which the long term problems of haemophilia can be prevented?

57 Are there any common drugs which haemophiliacs should avoid?

# D  Psychiatric and behavioural disorders

58  How common is insomnia as a presenting problem in general practice?

59  What should be your management of insomnia?

60  What are the problems associated with the use of hypnotics in the elderly?

61  What are the general principles of management of patients with an acute anxiety state?

62  What is the management of a dementing elderly patient in the community?

63  What are the signs and symptoms of depression occurring in an elderly patient?

64  Before starting a patient on tricylic antidepressants what are the important things to tell him?

65  What are the 'risk' factors for alcoholism?

66  What is the method for alcohol withdrawal from a patient in the community?

67  What is the management of 'school refusal'?

68  What is meant by the term, abdominal migraine?

69  What are the characteristics of breath-holding attacks in children?

70  Enuresis is a common childhood problem but how common is it?

71  How should we manage the enuretic child?

# E  Disorders of the nervous system

72  A mother of a young child states she thinks her child may be more than daydreaming. What is she worried about?

73  What do you consider to be occurring when a patient's wife states that her husband has

started 'wetting the bed' and complains of waking headaches?

74    What are the indications for the use of seizure prophylaxis in febrile children?

75    In epileptic adults what social aspects should be discussed?

76    What is a characteristic feature of chronic subdural haematoma in the elderly?

77    Should all head injuries which present to the doctor have a skull X-ray?

78    In the evaluation of headache and facial pain what is the most important point?

79    What are the characteristics of tension headaches?

80    What are the general principles of management of headache and migraine?

81    What is the specific treatment for migraine?

82    What are the presenting features of Parkinson's disease?

83    What are the principles of management of Parkinson's disease?

84    In checking for patients with dysphasia what is a simple test?

85    What is the management of acute vestibular failure?

86    What are the risk factors associated with cerebral infarction?

87    What are the aims of management of the acute stroke?

88    What are the complications of stoke?

89    What are the main ways in which cerebral tumours present?

90  What is the treatment of acute torticollis (wry neck)?

91  What is meant by the term 'carpal tunnel syndrome'?

92  What is the theoretical management of pain?

# F  Obstetrical problems and gynaecological disorders

93  What are the general principles relating to counselling a female patient for contraception?

94  What advice would you give to a lady for whom you were prescribing the pill for the first time?

95  How soon after childbirth may the oral contraceptive be prescribed?

96  What are the serious possible complications of the combined oral contraceptive?

97  In the following examples are problems of oral contraception. What are the appropriate solutions in each case?
    (a) A general feeling of bloatedness with breast discomfort and loss of libido.
    (b) Midcycle breakthrough bleeding with heavier periods.
    (c) First ever migraine attack.
    (d) Missed withdrawal bleeding in a patient on a low dose combined pill.

98  What are the groups of drugs which can reduce the efficiency of the pill by interaction and give one example of each?

99  What are the advantages of the intrauterine contraceptive device?

100  What are the characteristics of the premenstrual syndrome?

101  What are the regimens of treatment for premenstrual tension?

102  What are the common causes and appropriate management of deep dyspareunia?

103  What is the treatment of herpes genitalis in females?

104 What are the commonest causes of vaginal discharge in prepubertal girls?

105 What are the conditions that favour monilial infection in the vagina?

106 Which women should have cervical smears and how often should they be taken?

107 How should you manage a woman with menopausal symptoms?

108 What are the medical treatments for the symptoms of the menopause?

109 What is the management of a woman who is pregnant and believes she has been in contact with rubella?

110 Which drugs, if given in early pregnancy could possibly cause congenital malformations?

111 What are the benefits and disadvantages of home confinements?

112 If a mother discontinues breast feeding what are the possible reasons for her doing so?


## G Disorders of ear, nose and throat

113 What percentage of a general practitioner's workload is constituted by diseases of the ear, nose and throat?

114 What is the underlying cause of inflamed ears in childhood and what are the predisposing factors?

115 What is the management of acute otitis media in children?

116 What is the commonest cause of acute deafness and what is its management?

117 What is the management of a foreign body in a child's ear?

118 At what age can hearing be accurately tested and describe how it is carried out?

119 What is the treatment of otitis externa?

120 What is the management of Menière's syndrome during remission?

121 What is the commonest cause of vertigo presented to the general practitioner?

122 What are the characteristics of positional vertigo?

123 What is the management of acute vertigo?

124 What is the characteristic type of hearing loss sustained by workers subjected to constant loud noise?

125 What is the most effective treatment for tinnitus of unknown origin?

126 What are the three commonest causes of acute sore throat?

127 What are the indications for tonsillectomy?

128 What is the management of epistaxis in general practice?

129 What is the management of chronic rhinitis?

130 How long is it reasonble to wait for the spontaneous resolution of hoarseness?

131 What are the clinical features of Bell's palsy?

## H Disorders of the circulatory system

132 How do you diagnose angina pectoris?

133 What are the ways in which angina pectoris can present abnormally?

134 In a patient with known ischaemic heart disease what general dieting advice should be given?

135 What are the mainstays of treatment of angina pectoris currently available to general practitioners?

136 A common treatment of angina pectoris is

trinitrin tablets. What do you explain to a patient on initially giving them?

137 How vital is the role of the GP in the treatment of acute myocardial infarction?

138 What is the management of bradycardia after myocardial infarction?

139 In a patient who has had a myocardial infarction 3 weeks ago what does the sudden onset of shortness of breath signify?

140 What is the role of the exercise test in the management of coronary artery disease?

141 How soon after an acute myocardial infarction may a man have sexual intercourse?

142 In the general practice situation it is considered important to track down patients who have hypertension. How may this be carried out?

143 What are the aims of hypertensive management?

144 What are the general principles of management of hypertension other than drug therapy?

145 When checking if a patient is hypertensive what are the factors that can cause error?

146 What is the mainstay of treatment of cardiac failure?

147 What are the alternatives to a patient taking potassium supplements while on diuretics?

148 What are the risk factors predisposing to deep venous thrombosis?

149 In patients with leg ischaemia what precautions should you ask them to take?

150 What is the management of night cramps?

## I  Disorders of the respiratory system

151  What proportion of a GP's workload is due to respiratory illness?

152  How do you help someone who wishes to give up smoking?

153  Is there any evidence that some patients can have genetic resistance to cigarette smoking?

154  Why do patients with a cough present themselves to their general practitioner?

155  In a patient with hay fever what common sense advice can you give him?

156  What is the role of desensitization in the treatment of hay fever?

157  How would you instruct a patient in the use of a metered aerosol?

158  Should steroid inhalers be used continuously or only during acute exacerbations of bronchial asthma?

159  What are the general principles of management of a person with bronchial asthma?

160  In a patient with chronic obstructive airways disease what are the aims of management?

161  What are the early manifestations of acute respiratory insufficiency?

162  What are the features in the history and examination which suggests a non-bacterial pneumonia?

163  Are there any dangers in giving hypnotics to sufferers from chronic bronchitis or emphysema?

164  In an acute exacerbation of chronic bronchitis how much reliance should be placed on bacteriology reports?

165  What are the risk factors associated with chronic bronchitis?

166 What is the management of chronic bronchitis and what factors do you consider?

167 Are there indications for the use of $O_2$ in the home?

168 What clinical pointers would make you consider the diagnosis of bronchogenic carcinoma?

## J Disorders of the urogenital system

169 What proportion of general practitioners' workload is due to diseases of the genitourinary tract?

170 What are the benefits of microscoping urine in the surgery?

171 What steps would you take if a mother brought a preschool child with a urinary infection?

172 What is the management of a 3-year-old boy with a first attack of balanitis?

173 What is the management of urinary tract infection in adult men?

174 What are the predisposing factors leading to acute cystitis in adult women?

175 What is the management of women who suffer from frequent urinary tract infections?

176 If you find proteinuria on incidental 'stick' testing what do you do next?

177 What are possible causes of proteinuria other than renal disease?

178 Hypernephroma can present with the typical triad of loin pain, haematuria and abdominal swelling, but it is renowned for its obscure presentations. What are they?

179 Red urine is usually due to blood but occasionally there are other causes. What are they?

180 What is the ideal treatment for the gastrointes-

tinal symptoms which are common in patients with renal failure?

181    What are the areas of clinical management of chronic renal failure?

182    In a patient who has had renal transplantation explain the occurrence of widespread warts.

183    What are the most common causes of infection after vasectomy?

184    Is circumcision advisable in a 30-year-old male patient who experiences pain during intercourse associated with stretching and tearing of the frenum?

185    When discussing psychosexual problems how can you encourage patients to air their feelings?

186    If a married woman complains of vaginal itching after intercourse when a condom is not being used what is the likely cause?

187    Should any foods or drinks be avoided to minimize symptoms in a patient with mild prostatic hypertrophy?

188    How common a problem is incontinence in the elderly?


## K    Disorders of the skin

189    How commonly do skin diseases present in general practice?

190    When confronted with a dermatological problem on what areas of questioning do you concentrate?

191    What is the commonest cause of eczema in children? What are its features?

192    What is cradle-cap and how is it managed?

193    How do you manage napkin rash in babies?

194    What is the usual pathogenesis of a small red

spot which can appear on a baby's head or upper chest a few days after birth?

195   Sunlight is a recognized treatment for psoriasis. Why in some cases does it actually deteriorate in summer?

196   Dithranol is probably the mainstay of psoriasis treatment but what do you tell the patient about its use?

197   If a psoriatic using dithranol ointment develops soreness during the treatment what do you tell him?

198   What is the role of the strong steroid preparations in psoriasis?

199   What are the basic principles in the use of topical steroids?

200   Which skin lesions can be treated in general practice by the use of injected steroid preparations?

201   What is the management of someone who complains of severe under-arm sweating?

202   What is the management of juvenile acne vulgaris?

203   What are the indications that a naevus has become malignant?

204   What are the clinical features and treatment of a rodent ulcer?

205   Scaly red lesions on the feet can be caused by either fungal or psoriatic lesions. How is it possible to separate the two?

206   Erythema abigne is common in the elderly but what particular condition is associated?

207   What is the management of venous ulcers?

## L  Disorders of bones and joints

208  How common are rheumatic problems in general practice?

209  What are the principles of management of sports injuries?

210  What are the features of back strain which if present make the diagnosis of disc prolapse *unlikely*?

211  If a patient suffers from recurrent 'back troubles' what general advice do you offer to him?

212  When an acute meniscus tear is diagnosed is early operation by meniscectomy the treatment of choice?

213  Arthroscopy is becoming more widely available. What would be your reasons for recommending this investigation in one of your patients?

214  What are the special considerations regarding the use of drugs in the treatment of arthritic conditions?

215  Why is there such a narrow range of effectiveness for salicylic acid before toxicity occurs?

216  What are the principles of management of a patient you have decided to start on systemic steroids?

217  During an acute attack of gout should you treat the underlying hyperuricaemia?

218  What are the principles of management of a young person developing ankylosing spondylitis?

219  What is the value of a Westergren erythrocyte sedimentation rate (ESR) in patients with rheumatic sysmptoms?

220  What is the commonest presenting symptom of rheumatoid arthritis?

221 What are the presenting features of rheumatoid arthritis which indicate a poor prognosis?

222 Some patients are given gold injections for rheumatoid arthritis but what precuations should you take?

223 If a man of 50 years presents with a seronegative, and inexplicable arthropathy what single most important additional check should you make?

224 What are the principles of management of osteoarthrosis?

225 Disabled people suffer various social handicaps. What are these?

## M Disorders of the digestive system

226 How common are abdominal emergencies in general practice and what proportion of the total workload do they constitute?

227 What clinical pointers exist that indicate pathological jaundice in the first 2 weeks of life?

228 In patients with hiatus hernia syndrome and reflux, what are the indications for surgery?

229 Malnutrition is easily overlooked. What are the high risk groups in general practice?

230 What is the theoretical reason for avoiding antacids which contain calcium salts?

231 In patients with peptic ulceration what dietary advice would you give?

232 What is the management of bleeding from a suspected duodenal ulcer?

233 What are the clinical pointers which should make you suspect a gastric neoplasm?

234 What is it reasonable to expect a general practitioner to carry out in the follow-up of patients having had gastric surgery?

235    What advice would you give to a patient with a true dumping syndrome after partial gastrectomy?

236    What are the two most difficult aspects of management of patients with chronic pancreatitis?

237    When liver disease is suspected what initial investigations should you carry out?

238    Which kinds of viral hepatitis can lead to permanent liver damage?

239    When would you consider dissolution therapy for patients with gallstones?

240    What are the four main presentations of carcinoma of the large bowel?

241    What advice would you give to a patient to establish a normal bowel habit?

242    Which constipated patients should be referred for a second opinion?

243    How common is diverticulosis in the community and what general recommendations should you give to sufferers?

244    Why might Crohn's disease not be diagnosed in its early stages?

245    At what point would you refer a patient with Crohn's disease for a surgical opinion?

246    What is the management of ulcerative colitis in general practice?

247    What is the place of sulphasalazine in the treatment of ulcerative colitis?

248    What are the general principles of stoma care in the community?


N    Disorders of the eye

249    What proportion of a general practitioner's workload is constituted by diseases of the eyes?

250 What is the management of an acute corneal abrasion?

251 What is a 'welder's flash' and how is it managed?

252 Antiviral agents have one major limitation. What is it?

253 What is the mechanism of production of a dry eye?

254 What is a common cause of chronically red eyes in the elderly?

255 How frequently should eye drops be instilled in an eye to produce a cure?

256 What are the principles of treatment for styes and meibomian abscesses?

257 What are the hazards of prolonged corticosteroid therapy?

258 Many mothers bring children with eyes that appear to be squinting but turn out not to be on critical testing. Why is this so?

259 At what point should you advise a patient to have a cataract operation? And what is its effect?

260 Why should ladies who wear contact lenses be cautioned about taking the combined contraceptive pill?

261 How can you test visual activity in a patient who cannot read at all?

262 How can you test if a patient's deteriorating vision is due to poor correction by spectacles or due to macula degeneration?

263 What is braille?

## O Emergency situations in practice

264 What are the indications for hospital admission in a child with gastroenteritis?

265 After seeing a clinically shocked patient in the home and deciding to admit to hospital what advice would you give to the ambulance personnel?

266 What are the warning signs for child abuse being present?

267 How do you manage a patient with an acute confusional state?

268 What is the management of a patient with a panic attack seen in their home?

269 How should you manage a patient who makes a suicidal gesture?

270 How do you assess suicidal risk in a depressed patient?

271 What is the management of a child with a febrile illness and known to have had a previous febrile convulsion?

272 How would you manage a case of status epilepticus?

273 In a child with croup what are the factors which would result in a decision to admit to hospital?

274 How is it possible to overlook a case of acute myocardial infarction?

275 What is the indication for the use of lignocaine in the early treatment of myocardial infarction?

276 What are the factors that favour management of an acute myocardial infarction at home?

277 In a patient with acute pneumonia what are the indicators for management in hospital?

278 What are the danger signs in an acute asthmatic attack which would cause you to arrange urgent hospital admission?

279 In acute respiratory illness what features if developed would cause you alarm?

280    What are the clues that help identify a drug reaction?

281    What is the management of a patient with acute back pain?

282    What are the principles of management of foreign bodies which are extraocular?

283    What precautions do you take when a patient presents with a black eye?

284    What are the diagnostic symptoms of acute angle-closure glaucoma?

285    On what occasions must a patient's death be reported to the coroner?

# HUMAN BEHAVIOUR

286    What are the objectives for a consultation?

287    What is the importance of physical contact in the consultation?

288    What factors are important to how much information is retained by a patient after a consultation?

289    What are the common situations in which a patient may minimize his symptoms?

290    When might guilt feelings present in a consultation?

291    What do you understand by the term 'regression' when considering patients' behaviour in illness?

292    Reassurance in a consultation is extremely important but sometimes this measure fails. What are some common indications that a doctor's attempt at reassurance have failed?

293    What is the main danger of recognizing 'stress' as the underlying cause of physical symptoms?

294    What do the following situations have in common:

the menopause
death of a spouse
retirement
a teenager going to university
marriage?

295 What are the dangers of allowing aggressive behaviour to take place in a consultation?

296 What is meant by the term 'patient compliance'?

297 What are the possible social factors which can lead to marital breakdown?

298 What are the four main areas which should be enquired about when a patient presents with 'stress'?

299 What are the three levels of response to stress?

300 What are the typical stages of a grief reaction?

301 What are the predictors of a poor outcome to a grief reaction?

302 Describe in broad terms the characteristics of a large low income family?

303. How would you improve the communication between general practitioner, family, and hospital team when serious illness is diagnosed?

304 Which groups of drugs have a deleterious effect on driving?

## HUMAN DEVELOPMENT

305 What are the unique features of general practice which allow preventive care to be practised?

306 What are the objectives for child care in the community?

307 What are the occasions when immunization with live vaccines is contraindicated?

308 What are the contraindications to immunization with pertussis vaccine?

309 In a 6-month-old child what developmental milestones would you expect to be achieved?

310 What do you understand by the term percentile chart and what is its application?

311 How often is tongue-tie a cause of feeding difficulties?

312 What is the management of a child whose parent considers him to have an abnormal gait?

313 Should general practitioners make time to manage adolescent psychosexual behaviour?

314 What is the greatest difficulty in dealing with adolescent patients?

315 A worried mother brings her adolescent son saying that he is having 'wet dreams' and these normally happen once a week. What do you say to her?

316 If you were to set up a 'well-woman' clinic what areas would you assess?

317 What are the objectives of general practitioners for the care of their elderly patients?

318 In general terms what are the major problems of the elderly?

319 What is the extent of the geriatric problem in general practice?

320 What are the major problems in dealing with the terminally ill?

321 How do you tell a patient he has a terminal illness?

322 What are the services that can be provided by social services?

# THE PRACTICE AND PRACTICE ORGANIZATION

323 What are the strengths and drawbacks of an appointment system?

324 What are the basic components of a practice information system?

325 What are the basic requirements for a good medical record?

326 What are the principles underlying the entry of details of a consultation in the clinical records?

327 What register is an essential research tool? Describe its structure.

328 How would you compile an age/sex register?

329 How is the age/sex register used in research?

330 What are the most commonly prescribed drugs in general practice?

331 What are the requirements for an efficient repeat prescribing system?

332 If we accept that patient involvement improves 'compliance' how can we make use of this in the primary care situation?

333 What do you do if you suspect a patient has reacted to a prescribed drug?

334 In prescribing a 'controlled' drug under Schedule 2 of the Misuse of Drugs Act 1971 and Misuse of Drugs Regulations 1973 what must a general practitioner do?

335 What is the role of the attached local authority nurse in the primary care team?

336 What services does the Family Practitioner Committee (FPC) oversee?

337 What are the functions of the family practitioner committee in respect of general practitioners?

338 What are the terms of service of a general practitioner?

339 What is the range of disciplinary action which

the General Medical Council can take when a
doctor is found guilty of serious professional
misconduct?

340 When discussing a product with a pharmaceutical representative what points should you
check?

# 3
# Answers

## CLINICAL MEDICINE

### A Infective and parasitic diseases

1 The greatest danger in these children is dehydration and the degree must be assessed.

When moderate in severity then there is depression of the fontanelle, sunken eyes and loss of skin turgor. The child is usually lethargic and listless and may cry fitfully. These are indications for immediate fluid replacement. If oral fluids are refused or vomited back then parenteral fluids are indicated after hospital admission. The most satisfactory oral preparation is glucose and sodium chloride mixture. A proprietory combination is available.

If the child remains untreated then the degree worsens and a rapid weak pulse is detected with cold blue extremities. Fluid replacement is then an emergency procedure. In infants who have an excessive sodium intake, e.g. those fed on cows' milk in an unmodified form, then serious hypernatraemia may occur. In these cases there is insufficient water to excrete the sodium load and this can result in permanent neurological damage and twitching followed by fits is common. Water replacement is even more urgent in these cases.

2 The causative organism is a strain of group A haemolytic streptococci and the serious sequelae of rheumatic fever and acute glomerulonephritis are extremely rare. The incubation period is usually 3 days but can vary from 1 to 7 days. The patient complains of headache, sore throat, vomiting and has a coated tongue and rash. The symptoms are fleeting but a pyrexia of up to 40°C can be present for the first 3 days. The tonsils are enlarged, infected and covered with a white exudate. The rash usually appears on the second or occasionally the third day. It has the appearance of intensely red, punctate spots affecting the face, neck, chest, upper

27

trunk, arms and thighs—lastly spreading to the lower legs. The thick white coating on the tongue peels off on the 3rd or 4th day leaving a typically 'strawberry' appearance. The rash lasts several days and is followed by scaling, particularly on the hands. The patient should have a high fluid intake with salicylates for the fever. A 5 day course of penicillin eradicates the organism which is much less virulent than it was in previous years.

3 This virus infection commonly presents as an upper respiratory tract problem with fever lasting approximately 4–7 days. The child usually has pink watery eyes, is anorexic, miserable and lethargic. He is disturbed by a repetitive dry cough and when sought there are small 'grain of salt' type granules on the buccal mucosa opposite the molar teeth, in the early stages. These are known as Koplik's spots which appear on day 2 or 3 and approximately 24 hours prior to the full rash. The typical rash appears on the neck and spreads to the face, trunk and limbs. The early lesions are macules which eventually become maculopapular and finally confluent, leaving only small areas unaffected. Typical brawny staining then becomes evident when the rash has been present for up to 4 days. All the symptoms described above are due to viral involvement of those particular systems.

4 These are the tiny salt-grain-like lesions which are specific to measles and occur 24 hours or so before the typical erythematous rash. They are areas of necrosis on the buccal mucosa and can be seen on the inside of the cheek near the upper second molar and often on the gums at the front. The time to spot them is during the catarrhal phase of the illness.

5 In the early phase of merely contact with an infectious case then a 10 day course of erythromycin is advisable. In the established case antibiotics should be avoided. Erythromycin may be of value in the catarrhal phase, although this is unproven and ampicillin is the drug of choice for bronchopneumonia. The drug second on your list should be co-trimoxazole.

Antitussives are as usual ineffective but atropine methonitrate 0.6% in 90% alcohol can be useful. Some authorities advocate phenobarbitone as a sedative to diminish irritative factors that produce coughing spasms. Other authorities advocate beta-agonists such as salbutamol which are also thought to be beneficial.

In the occasional case of lung collapse or bronchopneumonia physiotherapy is helpful and this can be taught to the parents. Turning the child head down during coughing spasms prevents inhalation of secretions and vomit.

A full discussion with the parents regarding the course of the illness is especially important in regard to the protracted nature of the illness and it should be stressed that careful nursing during the spasms is important. Incidentally, one advantage of the use of routine erythromycin ensures that the child is no longer infective and may return to school as soon as coughing spasms permit.

6  No. The mode of transmission of chickenpox is by either direct, contact, droplet or airborne spread. Herpes zoster (shingles) is caused by reactivation of the virus which has remained dormant in the dorsal root ganglion after a previous attack of chickenpox, probably in childhood. Patients with shingles, however, can cause chickenpox to occur in susceptible individuals and the virus may be cultured from the lesions.

7  Ampicillin—this is because of the invariable production of a maculopapular rash which can be severe. Where a throat swab culture reveals beta-haemolytic streptococcus then phenoxymethylpenicillin is indicated or erythromycin in cases of penicillin allergy.

8  (a) The majority of cases begin with fever, anorexia, sweating and weight loss and commonly are initially diagnosed as having influenza as myalgia is prominent.
   (b) If the sputum when produced contains large numbers of pus cells, but no organisms on conventional staining then the index of suspicion should be high.
   (c) The patient is often confused and agitated (50% of cases).

(d) There is a fever with a temperature of 30–40.5°C with tachypnoea. Course râles are heard on auscultation and consolidation follows.

(e) There is no response to antibiotics unless erythromycin is used early in the course of the illness.

(f) The patient who is suffering already from an illness or is on therapy which is compromising their immune response is suspect.

9   Persuading the patient to continue taking the therapy. It is always difficult to motivate a patient to adhere to a complicated treatment regimen long after they feel better. Constant monitoring and follow-up is necessary. At each interview it is important to stress this and leaflets which the patient can take away and read are useful. The enthusiasm and interest of the doctor also has a profound effect. Here the doctor–patient relationship is important.

Don't forget that in many areas the immigrant population is a reservoir of infection and when treating this family an interpreter is often necessary and this also means your advice leaflets will need to be printed in the patient's language.

Modern chemotherapy is simple, well tolerated and effective. Among these are isoniazid, rifampicin and pyrazinamide. Remember of course drug interactions, a common one being rifampicin and the oral contraceptive.

With these modern regimens, cure can be attained in 6–9 months and this fact alone is encouraging to the patient, as most retain the concept that a cure will take years and may require admission to a sanitorium.

10   (a) It enables legal powers to be invoked in the case of outbreaks of disease in order to bring them under control.

(b) To provide data for monitoring infection both locally and nationally.

(c) Early attempts to control the spread of infectious disease can be organized providing early notification is carried out.

11   (a) Take a full and detailed history which should define the patient's itinerary, what immunization and other prophylactic pro-

cedures had been performed and whether they had been in contact with any other persons who had been ill. Make a note as to whether untreated water had been drunk.

(b) Examine particularly any system where symptoms are indicative, e.g. lymph glands, skin etc.

(c) Carry out preliminary investigations of a general nature: full blood count and ESR with differential white cell count; urine, for microscopy, glucose, protein and bile salts. Finally, examine a thick blood film. When suspect blood samples are sent to a laboratory they should be enclosed in 'hazard' bags.

(d) In many cases a simple diagnosis after the above have been carried out can be made. If more sinister illness is suspected or if some of the investigations point to an unusual cause, then the district community physician should be contacted. Another useful source of help is your local pathology laboratory. In many cases they are aware of areas of endemic illness in other countries and are more closely informed of patterns of disease abroad.

(e) Antibiotics or antimalarials should not be prescribed empirically. These may make diagnosis less feasible and delay cure.

(f) An urgent outpatient referral may be indicated and occasionally admission to a district general hospital (with suitable warnings) is the proper action to take. When social and clinical factors permit, then treatment at home is to be recommended as this will lessen the chances of transmission to other individuals.

12  Whenever possible midstream samples should be collected after careful cleansing of the external genitalia. It is important not to use disinfectants for two reasons. First, they contaminate the sample and can give false negative results and second, they can produce local sensitizing reactions on mucous membranes. Samples from infants can be taken using self-adhesive plastic bags and removed when sufficient has been collected. Specimens should ideally reach the laboratory promptly, because the bacteria will multiply and leucocytes will degenerate

when kept at room temperature. If allowed to remain at room temperature for longer than 3 hours then results are invalid.

In practice the storage period can be extended by storage in the refrigerator at 4°C, by dip-slides or spoons or the addition of boric acid which is a bacterial preservative. One useful and economical method is to run the midstream urine sample over a CLED slope in a sterile container immediately after the sample has been voided. CLED stands for Cysteine Lactose Electrolyte Deficient and this is a culture medium particularly suitable for coliform organisms. The container is then incubated for 24 hours in the surgery and only 'positive' results need be sent to the pathology laboratory for colony indentification and sensitivities.

13  The effect of a pathogen on phagocytes is to cause the release of endogenous pyrogen. The pyrogen acts on the thermoregulatory centre and information then is transmitted via local prostaglandin production to the vasomotor centre, i.e. turning up the thermostat. Heat generation is increased and heat loss prevented. e.g. by shivering. It should be noted that many different temperature patterns can be produced by any one disease and that a pattern may not be characteristic.

14  (a) The cause of the fever may not be bacterial in origin or even sensitive to that particular antibiotic.
    (b) The diagnosis may be confused due to the production of side effects or drug interaction, e.g. rashes, diarrhoea, vomiting etc.
    (c) The diagnosis in certain conditions may be masked by inadequate treatment or underlying pathology may not come to light, e.g. myocarditis, endocarditis.
    (d) The cost of the preparation is in some cases considerable and when multiplied by the number of general practitioners in the country the total drug bill is staggering.
    (e) The long term effect of using antibiotics in self-limiting illness is to place the stamp 'justifiable' on the patient's attendance. It is much better to initially spend longer with the patient, giving health education.

15  (a) An age–sex register or computer printout

32

of all children in the age group to be immunized.
(b) A health education programme to promote generally the value of immunization.
(c) Counselling for individual parents.
(d) A system for the administration of the vaccine.
(e) An effective means of recalling defaulters.
(f) The measurement of immunization uptake rates and feedback.

16  The most susceptible age is the under-fives, but clinical infection is usually in the under-threes. Typically the mother describes a picture of poor appetite, loss of interest in playing and a failure to gain weight. These features are worse at certain times and the child may be found to be flushed and have a moderate fever (up to 39°C) on such occasions.

Specific organ involvement by the larvae dictates more specific features which can include:
(a) splenomegaly and lymph gland enlargement.
(b) ocular lesions—seen only with a slit lamp.
(c) hepatomegaly with abdominal pain.
(d) lung involvement with an asthma-like picture.
(e) Other rare sites are the brain and the myocardium.

This disease should be considered in any child under 5 with failure to thrive and specific points such as the eating of earth by the child should be asked of the parents. A raised eosinophil count is indicative and an elevated IgE and IgM help to differentiate toxocariasis from other non-allergic causes of marked eosinophilia.

17  Apart from eradicating the total dog and cat population relatively simple measures are useful. It must be remembered that the most susceptible group are children under 5 years of age, but symptoms may only be obvious in those children under 3. The major reservoirs of infection are puppies and therefore deworming is the most effective single measure. The most quoted regimen involves deworming at 2 weeks of age and redosing twice at 2 week

33

intervals. Adult dogs should be dewormed annually.

Children should therefore be discouraged from handling puppies under 6 weeks old and the licking of children and adults by dogs and cats should be prevented. Ideally hands should be washed after stroking animals, but behaviour such as this is difficult to instil.

18 The only two common worms in the UK are threadworms (*Enterobius vermicularis*) and roundworms (*Ascaris lumbricoides*). The former, however, is the most common although rarer alternatives must be considered in immigrant communities. For most children, therefore, the only necessary investigation is taking of cellotape slides from the anus in the morning. It is necessary to treat the whole family at the same time to prevent reinfection. Analyses of epidemiology studies show peaks of infection at 5, 11 and 30 years. Recurrences in susceptible families are common and this suggests a reservoir of infection in untreated adults. The infective organism is white and thread-like and up to a centimetre long. The child usually complains of nocturnal itching and there may be visible excoriations. Treatment is usually with one of the piperazine compounds in doses related to age.

# B Endocrine disorders and disorders of metabolism

19 (a) To educate the individual as fully as possible within their capability as to the pathogenesis and management of diabetes. This will motivate the patient to give himself the best possible care and allow him to manage his own condition.
   (b) To correct to as near normal as possible the abnormal metabolic processes which are occurring.
   (c) To delay as much as possible the dangerous sequence of the condition and where possible prevent deterioration of the disease process. It has been shown that stabili-

zation of the blood glucose within the limits set down by the WHO significantly prevent complications.

20   (a) 'Juvenile' onset clinical diabetes, the normal time of onset being under 50 years of age, is insulin requiring.

     (b) 'Maturity' onset clinical diabetes, the onset usually being over 50 and initially controlled by diet alone or with the addition of oral hypoglycaemics.

     (c) Impaired glucose tolerance without symptoms or complications.

21   The principal use is in the elderly or type II diabetes when hyperglycaemia is present, but without ketonuria after about 4 weeks' treatment on a diabetic diet.

The two main kinds are biguanides and sulphonylureas. Of the former only metformin is used because of the problem of lactic acidosis.

Sulphonylureas such as glibenclamide are useful but there is always the danger of drug interaction. In addition profound hypoglycaemia can occur.

22   There are of course many reasons but the main are:

     (a) the aims and priorities are not adequately explained and the patient is not made aware of the importance of adhering to the diet.

     (b) the diet is not sufficiently related to the patient's eating habits. This is particularly a problem in immigrant communities advised by British doctors or dieticians.

     (c) educational facilities may be inadequate. Insufficient use may be made of literature, group instruction, audio-visual presentations.

     (d) many diet sheets are too complicated and the exchange list unnecessarily detailed.

     (e) differing advice given by different professions, e.g. dietician and doctor.

23   If you use beta-blockers to treat angina pectoris then glucose metabolism may be affected since this is also under the influence of the adrenergic system. If a diabetic becomes

hypoglycaemic then not only is this made more likely with beta-blockers, but the symptoms may be masked until the degree is marked. In addition the subsequent mobilization of glucose is slowed. In diabetics, therefore, cardioselective beta-blockers are to be preferred but caution must be exerted.

24  (a) Occupation—some occupations must be excluded from the list of possibilities open to young diabetics. For example insulin dependent diabetics are unable to hold a heavy goods vehicle or public service vehicle licence. Certain occupations involve irregular hours with on-call emergency needs and here the lack of routine is prohibitive. Altitude should be avoided when unprotected as intervening hypoglycaemia could be fatal.
   (b) Marriage—although the genetic transmission of diabetes is complex the possibility should be discussed. In females the possible problems in pregnancy are important and this point is usually debated before marriage is discussed, as it could affect marital relations.
   (c) Housing—because of the increased risk to life because of complications (mainly cardiovascular) insurance is more difficult to obtain and this can affect mortgage availability.

Diabetics, like many other groups of patients learn a great deal from others with similar problems. It is useful to refer them to the British Diabetic Association who have a comprehensive reading list. A local self-help group is a useful management tool and having an intelligent sensible young diabetic in the practice can be very helpful as an encouragement to others.

25  There are four major causes.
   (a) Thyrotoxicosis. In the young age group a woman with Graves' disease has heat intolerance, a good appetitie, excessive sweating, a fine tremor and complains of feeling agitated. In the elderly it is a much more difficult diagnosis to make, but atrial fibrillation is usually present along with cardiac

failure. In this age group it is the cardiovascular system which suffers most. Another symptom in the elderly is that they find it increasingly difficult to walk upstairs or hang up the washing. This is because the proximal muscle groups are involved, particularly the deltoid and the gluteals.

(b) Anorexia nervosa. Usually the patient is 'dragged' to the doctor by the mother or father. The patients look upon themselves as being of normal weight or even overweight. It is as if they have a distorted body image.

(c) Diabetes mellitus. Usually present in the adult with frequency, polyuria, polydipsia and weight loss in spite of a good appetite. An elevated blood sugar or the presence of glycosuria 3 hours after a meal is indicative and a glucose tolerance curve will prove the diagnosis. Only in adults does the picture often appear like this. In children hyperglycaemic coma is the presenting diagnosis. In the elderly general ill health or intercurrent infection is the norm.

(d) Addison's disease. Fatigue is usually the presenting feature and weight loss a secondary consideration.

26  Thyrotoxicosis in adults is typified by the presence of a hot sweaty skin. This is due to the body attempting to increase heat loss. In the case of anxiety neurosis there is hyperadrenalism with consequent pale cool skin which is clammy due to non-evaporation of sweat. The anxious patient also tends to have a previous history of nervous instability while for the organic thyrotoxic patient it is usually out of character. Finally, the thyrotoxic patient loses weight in spite of a normal or increased appetite. In patients with an anxiety state it is normal that they can not settle to eat a proper meal.

It is less than fair when a neurotic patient becomes thyrotoxic.

27  An urgent differential white cell count. All antithyroid preparations have agranulocytosis as a side effect in 1 patient in a 1000. Often the first symptom is a sore throat and a white cell count is diagnostic. If the drug is stopped then

normal white cells reappear within 3 weeks, but umbrella cover with a broad spectrum antibiotic is advisable during the waiting phase. Side effects of antithyroid drugs usually only take place in the first 3 months of therapy.

28  Yes. All therapy of this kind should be gradually introduced but in the elderly it should be excessively slowly. The reason for this is the load on the cardiovascular system since myocardial ischaemia can be induced. In addition it is possible to precipitate psychotic behaviour which can be reversed by stopping treatment and after a 'washout' phase, restarting but in an even more gradual way.

29  Instead of multi-system presentations as in the younger group, the most common presentation of hyperthyroidism in the elderly is in a single system. Cardiovascular symptoms and signs are the commonest perhaps, beause of the coexistence of ischaemic heart disease. Unexplained tachycardia persisting after standard diuretic therapy for heart failure of intermittent atrial fibrillation should alert you to the possibility of an overactive thyroid. Thyrotoxicosis may cause systolic hypertension. Atrial fibrillation associated with thyrotoxicosis in older people is more likely to revert to sinus rhythm after treatment than when it is due to cardiac ischaemia.

30  Fewer than 1% of obese patients have an organic cause, but when present they are as follows:

(a) hypothyroidism—most of the gain here is due to fluid retention, the deposition of fat and mucopolysaccharides. Their appearance is typical with coarseness of skin and loss of hair and a deepening of the voice.
(b) Cushing's syndrome—the typical picture here is a person with plethoric facies, obese thorax and abdomen and thin arms and legs. Purple striae are common but rapid weight gain from any cause may be responsible.
(c) hypogonadism—common in cases of delayed puberty and also Klinefelter's syndrome.

(d) polycystic ovaries syndrome—along with obesity the patient complains of amenorrhoea and hirsutes.

31  Before treatment can begin it is important that the patient be willing to lose weight. This is assumed in adults because they actually present themselves for advice. In children it is often the parents who bring along an unwilling child. The first task is to increase motivation. The most important single factor is the enthusiasm of the doctor and his willingness to give long term advice and support. A deep understanding of this is important in general practice as emotional and physical problems commonly are associated with 'simple' obesity. Many doctors find obese people unattractive and have trouble sympathizing with their problems. These attitudes contribute to the frequent lack of success in treating obese patients.

During the early phase of treatment it is important that the doctor should understand the feelings of the patient and he can improve motivation by emphasizing how well the patient will feel when he reaches the target weight. It is important to set a realistic target weight which can be calculated from an age/height/weight/sex chart. From this a rate of weight loss can be suggested. It is usually best to restrict calories by no more than 500–1000 per day below maintenance levels.

Two phases of weight loss occur on any diet. Initially fluid loss occurs as the body adjusts to using stored fats. After this the body adapts to caloric restriction by reducing caloric expenditure. This must be carefully explained to avoid frustration in the patient.

Close supervision and encouragement during this phase is paramount. Group therapy scores highly in this respect and it is exemplified by such an organization as Weight Watchers. In the surgery a special clinic can be set up using the knowledge of an attached health visitor and group attendance can be organized.

The nature of the diet varies from one area to another, underlining the fact that no perfect diet exists. To be successful it should be tailored to the patient's mental ability, occupation, dietary likes and dislikes, and economic status.

Drugs are controversial but on the whole are to be discouraged. In the long term the patient will be more self-reliant if no drugs are used and will not associate future weight gain with the need to revisit his general practitioner.

Exercise is useful in improving well-being and is to be encouraged. Unfortunately, there is also an increase in appetite. Less usual methods such as jaw-wiring and surgery are not used in general practice.

32   Prior to the onset of menstruation amenorrhoea is by definition present. With the onset of fertilization of the ovum menses cease. The presence of menstruation up to the first 12 weeks of pregnancy, however, is not uncommon. This is due to the fact that the developing ovum does not occupy the whole of the uterus and fluctuations of a sequential nature cause seemingly normal menses.

During lactation menses are also absent and may last for the whole time that breast feeding is taking place.

With the coming of the climacteric then the menopause occurs. The average age now for the cessation of menses is 51 years.

33   The first sign is enlargement of the testes which occurs on average about $11\frac{1}{2}$ years of age. Approximately one year later there is development of pubic hair which is on either side of the penis. At first it does not have the full male distribution. The third stage is penile enlargement which on average occurs a further year later at about $13\frac{1}{2}$ years. Around this time there is a growth spurt, which reaches its peak velocity at about 14 years of age.

34   There are two major groups of symptoms.

(a) The patient, who is almost always elderly, complains of bone pain particularly in the spine. This is of a chronic nature and of gradual onset. Progressive change in shape of the spine is common and may be due to degrees of compression fracture.

(b) Sudden onset of severe pain is associated with fractures in three areas:

40

    (i) vertebral body collapse is associated with pain maximal at the site of the lesion but may radiate around the trunk. It is aggravated by bending and sitting and easier when lying. Typical wedge fractures are seen on lateral X-ray.

    (ii) lower forearm fractures are common after mild trauma.

    (iii) a fracture of the femoral neck.

35 Infertility is a problem for both husband and wife and it is vital that the couple be investigated, rather than one member first. Infertility consultations are charged with tension and anxiety and often guilt. It is therefore the role of the GP to discuss and investigate sensitively and discreetly. Management therefore should be of the couple's situation rather than one partner's problem. Joint consultations when possible are helpful, especially in exploring the psychological implications. Separate consultations are necessary to investigate medically and allow confidential disclosures. In no circumstances should one partner be given details of the other's condition or result of investigations without permission.

36 The over-riding consideration here is that the patient himself, or equally common now, herself, should realize that he has an alcohol problem. The vast majority at first have little insight or personal honesty and feel that they could stop if they wanted to at any time. The realization should come to them ideally in such a way that they themselves desire treatment. Many consultations may be necessary and it is essential that the alcoholic should be allowed to explain how he feels and give the story of what causes him to drink heavily. It is within this history that lie the clues to treatment.

It is often necessary to involve other members of the patient's family, but the confidentiality of the patient must be observed and his permission sought.

Often the precipitating factor for the initial consultation is some form of emergency. The common ones are:

withdrawal tremor,
loss of occupation,
breathalysed by the police,

act of unaccustomed violence on the spouse or children.

Frequent appointments and a commitment to long term support are essential features of management.

The use of tranquillizers such as diazepam or Heminevrin in the early tremulous stage is helpful, but these should be withdrawn after a few weeks.

Self-help groups such as Alcoholics Anonymous can be very helpful, but usually the patient is reluctant to make contact in the early phase, but can be encourged to do so later.

High potency vitamins in the early phase improve well-being and reduce tremor in some cases. Most authorities believe their major value is to encourage the alcoholic to attend regularly for 'treatment'.

Drugs, such as Abstem and Antabuse have little place since a reformed alcoholic does not need them and a defaulter simply doesn't take the tablets. Unfortunately, the success rate is low, but the enthusiasm of the practitioner and the amount of support given significantly affects the outcome.

37  Alcohol-induced (fasting) hypoglycaemic coma can follow on imperceptibly from alcoholic stupor and is fatal in 45% of children and 10% of adults. It generally follows 6–18 hours after the ingestion of a moderate to large amount of alcohol. The cause is inhibition of gluconeogenesis by alcohol in a susceptible subject. Malnourishment is a contributory factor, but children are particularly affected. Glucagon is ineffective in elevating the blood sugar level and intravenous glucose is the recommended treatment. Hydrocortisone is also given in the severe cases.

Diagnosis is easy when the possibility is considered. A Dextrostix blood sugar reading is all that is required, but failure to recognize the cause of the coma and institute treatment leads to irreversible brain damage.

38  Alcoholism. Excessive alcohol intake can appear almost identical to Cushing's disease, both clinically and biochemically. It is ex-

tremely important to be aware of this and take a careful history of alcohol intake and note the occupation of the patient. A serum glutamyl-transferase is diagnostic. Cessation of alcohol causes the signs and symptoms to revert to normal.

39  (a) Patients from families of social class 4 and 5 are much less common than from 1 and 2. However, when they occur the outlook is more serious.
    (b) Males are less common than teenage girls, but the anorexic male is usually severe and often intractable.
    (c) When a patient comes from a family where dieting and weight control is obsessional then relapses are more frequent.
    (d) Pre-morbid obesity or Bulimia nervosa worsen the prognosis.
    (e) A poor or immature personality causes greater chronicity.
    (f) If the parents are prone to psychiatric out-bursts and or marital breakdown then this has a detrimental effect on the patient.
    (g) The longer it takes for the initial episode to settle then the greater the risk of recurrence and the poorer the long term prognosis.

## C  Diseases of blood and blood-forming organs

40  Recent work has shown the variation to be much greater than previously believed. The upper limit of normal can be determined with the following simple formulae.

$$\text{Men} = \frac{\text{age in years}}{2}$$
$$\text{Women} = \frac{\text{age in years} + 10}{2}$$

41  The signs of anaemia include pallor of the skin and mucosae and also the conjunctivae. In hae-molytic anaemia, jaundice is frequently present. The cardiovascular consequences of anaemia may also be evident ranging in sever-ity from congestive cardiac failure with oedema, venous and pulmonary congestion to increased cardiac output with tachycardia on

rest or mild exertion accompanied by systolic flow murmurs. Severe anaemia can lead to hypoxic vascular changes in the fundus with haemorrhages and exudates. Obviously the incidence of the findings depends on the severity and acuteness of onset and there is increasing severity when the anaemia is accompanied by other changes in the blood structure. In addition there are physical signs associated with the underlying cause of the anaemia, e.g. petechiae, telangiectasia etc.

42  Many patients in general practice believe themselves to be anaemic and one of the most usual requests is for the patient to put out their tongue. This, of course, is mainly to detect pallor but if glossitis is noticed then this is another aid to diagnosis. Painless glossitis occurs in 35–45% of patients suffering from iron deficiency anaemia.

43  (a) Ensure that iron deficiency truly exists before embarking on a programme of replacement.
     (b) Look for a cause of the iron deficiency and correct whenever possible.
     (c) Replace the iron stores by medication.
     (d) Follow up the patient adequately and make sure he returns to normal, and afterwards to replace the stores. It is important that the patient should know the reasons for all these in order to gain his cooperation.

44  Ferrous sulphate B.P. In order to correct anaemia a patient will need to absorb 15–30 mg of elemental iron per day and this can be derived from 100–200 mg of the ferrous compound per day. It is not necessary to use ascorbic acid to aid absorption as large amounts would be necessary and it is wasteful to use preparations with additives such as folic acid unless their deficiency has been proven.
       Ferrous sulphate is as good as any and cheaper than most and in a dose of 200 mg twice daily it is more than adequate. Enteric-coated or slow release preparations are used mainly to improve patient tolerance by reducing the number of tablets taken and the incidence of unpleasant gastrointestinal side effects in susceptible individuals. The majority

of the gastrointestinal side effects can be reduced by taking the preparations with food and for the first week or two by only taking one tablet per day.

45 There are three main reasons.

(a) The patient may have had iron previously and suffered gastrointestinal side effects.
(b) A common belief is that injections produce a much quicker response and therefore the improvement will be more rapid. The difference is in fact negligible after 24 hours.
(c) Because of the prolonged therapy course the patient fears forgetting to take the medication or indeed simply wishes to complete the treatment course as rapidly as possible and with little concentration from him.

The major dangers of parenteral iron and therefore your most useful argument towards persuading him to accept oral therapy are the possible reactions:

(a) GENERAL—anaphylactic response. To help reduce this risk small test doses should be given in closely supervised conditions.
(b) LOCAL reactions particularly in the form of pain and tissue staining.

46 There are four major causes.

(a) The most likely cause is failure to take the prescribed medication either because of side effects or just forgetfulness.
(b) Malabsorption.
(c) Incorrect diagnosis.
(d) Blood loss continuing to occur and the replacement being inadequate.

The complete case must be reviewed and a further careful history taken, and in most cases reinvestigation.

47 This is an emergency and admission to hospital is mandatory. While awaiting your arrival and providing it is now less than 2 hours since the child swallowed the tablets, ask the mother to give the child a glass of water containing fruit

juice and a tablespoon-full of salt. The latter is an emetic and the juice is to make the drink more palatable. When the vomiting has occurred or if the ingestion of iron took place longer than 2 hours prior to the phone call, instruct mother to give a mixture of raw eggs and milk. This inhibits iron absorption and binds the iron in the gastrointestinal tract.

Tell mum to try and act calm as this will help the child's behaviour and make him more likely to take the offered drinks. Arrange for the admission of the child as soon as possible. Explain the situation to mother and tell her to expect a gastric washout will be necessary for her child and perhaps intravenous therapy with desferrioxamine.

If it is impossible for you to attend quickly then arrange for immediate transfer to your local district general hospital by ambulance or by car if this is available. It is advisable for mum not to drive because she is likely to be in a very anxious state.

48  Iron deficiency anaemia. Most rheumatoid arthritics are taking medication of the anti-inflammatory analgesic type. This group of drugs which includes aspirin, phenylbutazone and indomethacin are prone to cause acute erosions which occur at the site of contact of particles of these drugs with the gastric mucosa. The effect is chronic blood loss leading to compensation on the part of the marrow. Eventually iron stores are depleted and clinical hypochromic anaemia results.

49  In the long term follow-up of patients suffering from PA there are three conditions to which they are more prone than the general population.

(a) Gastric carcinoma occurs approximately three times more commonly in PA patients than in the general population.

(b) Myxoedema—PA is a condition where autoantibodies are common (90% cases) and other autoimmune diseases are more commonly associated. The commonest of these is Hashimoto's disease the end result of which is myxoedema.

(c) Iron deficiency anaemia can intervene in PA as the atrophic gastritis can cause

46

microscopic and macroscopic blood loss and eventually stores are depleted.

50    The principle of replacement therapy is that more than the bare minimum is necessary to prevent symptoms. In this case, however, the feeling of tiredness is not due to B12 deficiency if the dose of hydroxycobalamin 1000 μg is given every 3 months. It is important to cover this aspect of patient education at the beginning of therapy and thus prevent misconception. If symptoms persist then another source of the tiredness must be looked for, although in these cases they are often psychogenic.

51    Alcoholism. The ethyl alcohol has a direct toxic effect on the marrow and confirmation of your suspicion can be made by checking the gamma GT level. Normally the macrocytosis will disappear within a few weeks of discontinuing the alcohol, but persistence indicates either a resumption of drinking or an accompanying nutritional folate deficiency. Apparently this is more common in spirit drinkers because of the 'purity' of the product.

52    ITP is primarily a disease of children and young adults and usually severity increases with age. In the elderly ITP is relatively unusual and is most commonly due to drugs. The most implicated compound is quinine bisulphate which is taken for night cramps. Since this symptom is a feature of many elderly patients then the result is predictable.

53    The general public believe that leukaemia is fatal especially in children. Mothers consider this diagnosis if their child is generally unwell and complains of lassitude. If easy bruising is also present along with pallor then their fears are heightened. The three classical signs of leukaemia are anaemia, easy bruising and lymphadenopathy. If these are present then it is obvious that further discussion and investigation are necessary.
   It is often the case that mothers will not directly mention their fears and it is important that you should check what they as parents believe to be wrong. It is a simple thing to ask 'Is there anything you are particularly worried

about?' or 'Have you any particular thoughts about it?'. It is important for you to say why you think it isn't leukaemia if all the characteristic features are not present. This does show that you have checked the possibility and it can help allay parent fears.

54 Because of the effect on the immune response by immunosuppressive therapy parents should be carefully counselled prior to any immunization programme. The body has a severely retarded ability to manufacture antibody to live vaccines and these can be fatal. The two most important are measles and poliomyelitis vaccines and previously smallpox. To give these is tantamount to injecting the lethal non-attenuated virus. Diphtheria and tetanus toxoids may be given as normal.

55 CLL is at present probably incurable but in most cases the disease lasts several years and can regress for long periods. It is important to discuss the condition with the patient in terms which are equivalent to his intellectual ability. If the diagnosis is in doubt or you or the patient's relatives don't believe he should be fully informed of the truth then alternative titles for the condition can be used.

In many instances no immediate therapy is necessary. However, bone marrow failure may be imminent or autoimmune haemolysis may be occurring in which case cytotoxic drugs are indicated.

Corticosteroids in high dosage can cause a dramatic reduction of lymphocyte mass but a side effect is to reduce resistance to infection.

Radiotherapy is useful in localized lymphadenopathy and symptoms due to splenomegaly can be treated in this way.

When the illness is resistant to all therapy then regular blood transfusions can be valuable.

Bactericidal antibiotics should be used in the early stages of bacterial illness. These have to be used blind as cultures cannot be awaited. In some cases prophylactic antibiotics are used. Human immunoglobulin is of debatable benefit and its effectiveness has not been evaluated.

56 The most important factor in preventing prob-

lems is for the patient to be thoroughly conversant with the pathogenesis of the disease. Naturally the intelligence of the patient determines the amount or type of knowledge to be imparted, but in the average case it is reasonable for a full description to be given in lay terms. There is no place for saying, 'You are an easy bleeder' and leaving it at that. The patient must appreciate what symptoms are serious and what kind of injuries can lead to trouble. Most medical problems relate either directly or indirectly to trauma and weight-bearing joints are most affected.

It is vital that prior to surgical and dental procedures factor VIII be given prophylactically to prevent coagulation problems.

57   One of the commonest symptoms which a haemophiliac will experience is joint pain. The temptation is to take aspirin and aspirin-containing preparations as these are readily available off prescription and do not require a visit to a doctor. The problem then is of course that aspirin damages platelet function through its effect on cyclo-oxygenase in the platelet prostaglandin pathway. Platelet adhesion is thereby impaired in someone already with a coagulation problem.

## D   Psychiatric and behavioural disorders

58   The consultation rate is 13.8 patients per 1000 population per annum, although there is a wide regional variation. It is commoner in females of all ages, but particularly in the elderly. Previous personality charcteristics play a large part.

59   (a) It is important to take a careful history and define any exacerbating factor causing insomnia. The causes are numerous and fall into five main areas:
(i) emotional stress by bereavement,
(ii) psychogenic disease, e.g. schizophrenia,
(iii) physical discomfort, e.g. pain,
(iv) drug abuse, e.g. alcohol,
(v) idiopathic.
(b) Explain the normal characteristics of sleep and the changes which occur with advancing age. Reassure that a lessening demand for sleep is common in the elderly.

(c) Give reassurance that loss of sleep at least for short periods is not harmful and usually self-limiting.

(d) Give advice to avoid stimulating activities before going to bed. It is better not to read too exciting a book before retiring or to enter into an argument. A warm (caffeine-free) drink can be recommended and a relaxing book.

(e) A reasonably fixed bed-time is to be commended as a routine is then developed.

(f) Regular physical exercise is to be advised especially in the evening.

(g) Forbid the taking of caffeinated drinks after 4 pm, e.g. coffee, tea, Lucozade and also alcohol especially in those with nocturia.

(h) In the short term, hypnotics such as benzodiazepines are helpful and break the vicious circle. Their temporary use should be emphasized and their long term side effects stressed.

60 (a) Dependence easily develops with continued use and this can be both physical and psychological. Naturally this makes withdrawal that much harder and a reduction in dosage must be made extremely slowly.

(b) When used in normal adult dosage they can cause confusion, agitation and a tendency to fall. Milder, shorter acting drugs should be substituted and gradually withdrawn, e.g. chlormethiazole and temazepam.

(c) The long term effect is a gradual deterioration in performance which heightens the normal dementing process. Explanation of this feature can help persuade a patient to stop.

61 Moderate degrees of anxiety are fairly commonplace e.g. prior to mixing with strangers, going to the doctors or even discussing money matters with a spouse. Patients should be encouraged to tolerate these as being normal. A thorough discussion of the problem and an appreciation that the doctor understands is often therapeutic.

Anxiolytic drugs should ideally not be prescribed at the first visit as it is more important that the patient should appreciate that the problem has been understood and should perhaps be allowed to generate his own solution. A diary should be kept by the patient and the times of anxiety should be noted and other concomitant features recorded e.g. two cups of strong coffee drunk, children arriving home from school etc. Explanation of these trigger factors is important and can be curative.

When necessary, the shorter acting benzodiazepines are to be preferred and their intermittent use recommended rather than regular dosage. It is important to stress that they are for temporary use only.

Non-drug treatments are acceptable in some patients and include such things as relaxation, meditation, yoga and hypnosis.

62  (a) Assess the degree of dementia and the rate at which it has progressed. If it is of recent onset then there is often an organic cause often of an infective nature. Afebrile chest and urinary infections are common and prompt treatment can reverse the dementia. Be especially wary if the patient is on steroids.

Underlying psychiatric disease such as depression or schizophrenia when treated can produce remarkable results.

Non-infective organic illness can also be present, particularly coronary artery disease, diabetes mellitus and temporal arteritis.

(b) Full active use of the primary care team is important to keep the patient in his home environment. Frequent visits by the practice health visitor or psychiatric social worker are helpful.

(c) Assess carefully the ability of the patient to manage at home balancing carefully the patient's feelings and the risk to his person.

(d) Involve the department of social services so that assessment for supervised accommodation can be made and arranged when necessary.

(e) Beware of complicated therapeutic regimens as these are unlikely to be complied with.

63  Occasionally bizarre symptoms can present themselves in the elderly and either anxiety or depression can be prominent. In some cases

the anxiety is expressed as agitation and over-activity and when stress occurs they simply 'go to pieces'. At the other end of the scale there is a feeling of 'couldn't care less' and their behaviour may be demanding in the extreme on close relatives, doctors and other primary care staff. They complain of being unable to cope and feel their confidence has disappeared. Normally outgoing individuals become socially withdrawn and fail to turn up at social gatherings, day care centres etc. They often complain of minor unassociated illnesses and paranoia may be a prominent symptom. Testing for memory loss is usually positive, especially for recent memory whilst distant memory frequently remains unimpaired. Typical characteristics are those of fairly recent personality change in someone who has previously been self-reliant.

64 (a) That the antidepressant effect will probably not start for 2 or 3 weeks, but that this is normal for all patients.
   (b) To expect anticholinergic side effects in all cases although these are not always significant and vary depending partly on previous personality and degree of neuroticism.
       It is usual for the patient to complain of a dry metallic taste in the mouth and if not present to doubt patient compliance. In the case of elderly males caution them about difficulties in micturition.
   (c) That the treatment course will be for several months after symptomatic recovery as stopping the drug prematurely increases significantly the risk of recurrence.
   (d) Treatment will commence with a low single daily dose taken at night and this will be progressively increased.
   (e) Regular supervision is necessary in the early stages. This allows smaller quantities to be prescribed and reduces the risk of overdosage as well as supporting the patient during the especially vulnerable phase.

65 There are two main groups.

   (a) Social. Marital disharmony and break-up; history of the alcoholism or heavy drinking in the family; occupation associated with

alcohol such as publican or hotelier or dray-
man; occupational boredom such as
seamen and unemployed; known original
tendencies; elderly single male; poor work
record.

(b) Medical. Peptic ulceration or 'indigestion';
chronic pancreatitis; cardiomyopathy; late
onset epilepsy; chronic psychiatric illness
involving frequent visits to the doctor; attempted suicide; recurrent minor accidents
either in the home or on the road.

66  The confusional state occurring during the
withdrawal of alcohol presents as an intense
fear that something is about to happen. There
is a marked tremulousness and sometimes
visual hallucinations. Withdrawal hypoglycaemic fits may occur and these should be
watched for.

The patient must want treatment as patient
cooperation is the most important factor. If
there is frank delirium tremens then hospital
admission is usually necessary. If the patient is
to be treated at home then the whole family
should be involved and their active cooperation
sought. First alcohol must be completely withdrawn and the tremor can in part be treated
with chlormethiazole 1 g four times a day. In
addition high dose vitamin B complex injections may be given especially if general nutrition has been poor.

The most important single factor is good
support by the family doctor or similar visitor.
This will mean very frequent visiting at first. As
time goes on the visits can be more spread out
and the chlormethiazole reduced.

67  This is a condition where children and parents
are implicated. First of all the condition must be
recognized and discussed between all members
of the family. Somatic symptoms if present
should be aired but unless the story is one of
obvious illness then very little investigation
should take place for not only will this be
fruitless but will serve to underline the organic
nature of the complaint.

There should be a careful enquiry into whatever complaints about school the child may
have. These often turn out to be significant but
not sufficient cause for school refusal, in that

the unpleasant experience has been a precipitating factor which summates with predisposing neurotic elements in the patient and the family.

Efforts should be made to correct such factors as inappropriate placement in school or class, educational backwardness, unnecessary sport, terrorism by older children etc.

Early return to school is essential and a firm date fixed. Parents should be reassured about the absence of physical disease. Getting a father involved whenever possible is a support for mother, who is usually left to struggle alone.

It is usually beneficial to involve social services and educational departments and their individual officers can be very supportive.

Minor tranquillizers may be helpful in the short term to reduce anxiety within bearable limits. A single morning dose of diazepam is all that is necessary.

In older children there may be frank psychiatric disease and depression of mood; loss of appetite and weight loss are important pointers to this. Such cases require appropriate therapy with major tranquillizers or tricyclic antidepressants.

68  This is a term sometimes used misleadingly as a synonym for recurrent abdominal pain. Only a small minority of children with recurrent abdominal pain develop classical migraine and there seems, therefore, no virtue in using the word until classical symptoms, i.e. headache of a unilateral nature preceding visual disturbance and vomiting, actually develop. The use of the term 'migraine' may have the disadvantage of allowing over-reacting parents the opportunity to label their children with an illness. The advantage of using such a simple descriptive term as 'recurrent abdominal pain' is that it helps to reduce the risk of overdramatization.

In over 90% of cases the pains are emotional or psychogenic in origin. Causes are more likely to be elucidated by enquiring into the family relationships and the social, emotional and educational aspects of the child's life. The important factor is to reassure the parents about the non-serious nature of the condition and the probable psychogenic cause. Treatment should be directed towards reassurance for the child and simple analgesics if necessary. In many cases the story of pain occurring during the school day rather than at weekends helps demonstrate to the parents the non-organic nature of the condition.

69 They are short episodes of unconsciousness which can be voluntarily induced in children under 3 years. Attacks are often precipitated by emotional upset or accidents. Typically the child holds his breath for a few seconds, then goes blue and limp for 30–60 seconds. Twitching can sometimes occur and the child may be markedly pale on recovery. The diagnosis rests on the mother's story. It is important to exclude major epilepsy.

70 The large majority of children are dry during the waking hours by the age of 3 years and dry at night by 4 but 10% of 5 year olds are enuretic, 5% of 10 year olds are enuretic and 10% of children of 4 years of age and older with a continuing problem have a urinary infection. If this is treated then 50% are cured.

With an average list size of 2400 patients a general practitioner will see 20 cases per year.

71 In the great majority of cases childhood enuresis is due to the development delay associated with a normal distribution curve. Approximately 10% of children are normally enuretic at 5 years of age.

It is important to take a careful history. If the child has never been dry then it is likely to be due to delayed development. If the child was once dry and has become wet then carefully explore all the important events around the time when the enuresis restarted. Often there was the birth of a sibling or perhaps a hospital admission of one member of the family. A physical examination and MSU culture will exclude a neurogenic bladder or urinary tract infection.

Initial therapy must involve explanation and strong reassurance. Simple behaviour techniques such as star charts and rewards are then used with counselling regarding restriction of fluids after 4 pm and 'lifting' the child when the parents go to bed. The next stage is the use of tricyclics, e.g. amitryptiline, which probably work via their effect on the bladder rather than their central effect on the brain.

The enuretic alarm buzzer is effective but can waken the whole household. It depends on the principle that the first few drops of urine complete a weak electric circuit and trigger the alarm buzzer.

# E   Disorders of the nervous system

72   The diagnosis in mother's mind is petit mal epilepsy. Since petit mal is brief and daydreaming is not, then the distinction is therefore involving the much rarer bird of status petit mal.

The other reassuring and distinguishing point is that a daydreaming child can be raised at any time. This is not so with petit mal.

73   Very frequently maturity onset grand mal epilepsy begins with nocturnal seizures and these are typified by loss of sphincter control and post-attack headache. Any history such as this requires full investigation including skull X-ray, EEG and CT scanning when available.

74   Phenobarbitone or sodium valproate are the drugs of choice in weight related dosage. The indications are:

(a) if the initial seizure is complex.
(b) if there is a family history of epilepsy.
(c) if the initial seizure occurred at less than 2 years of age.
(d) if there is pre-existing abnormality.
(e) if the child has had at least two seizures associated with fever.

Prophylaxis must be continuous to be effective. It is pointless giving phenobarbitone only at the time of the fever as it will take a week to attain adequate brain levels.

75   (a) A full explanation of the condition should be given and the patient encouraged to live a normal life.
(b) Hobbies. He should be encouraged to take exercise of all sorts, although he may only swim in the presence of a fellow swimmer

who is a life saver. All other exercises including team sports, rock-climbing etc. are allowable.

(c) A driving licence may be granted to an applicant who has suffered or is suffering from epilepsy if he has been free from any epileptic attack while awake for at least 2 years or in the case of an applicant who has had such attacks while asleep during that period he shall have been subject to such attacks while asleep but not while awake since before the beginning of that period. He may never drive a heavy goods vehicle or a public service vehicle.

(d) All jobs are open to him except those where a fall or disturbance of consciousness would be dangerous to himself or others, e.g. scaffold erecting. He cannot be recruited to the army, the police and usually not medicine. Many patients do not tell their employers as they fear dismissal. It is better if the employer knows and accepts the problem.

(e) Marriage. A future spouse must be informed as not to do so is grounds for annulment.

(f) Where there is a family tendency to epilepsy it may be transmitted, but it is rare for this to be direct from parent to the child.

(g) Pregnancy increases the tendency to fits and increasing the dosage of antiepileptics may be necessary temporarily. Breast feeding can still be recommended as little drug is transmitted and secreted in the milk. It is important that the epileptic mother should not bathe her baby alone.

(h) The oral contraceptive pill is not recommended in the usual small dosage. A 50 mg dosage of oestrogen should be given. There is no evidence that convulsions are commoner with this regimen.

(i) Several safety measures should be advised including the wearing of a warning identity bracelet or necklace. Around the home it is important to protect fires and staircases.

76 At first dementia is suspected but the classical picture is an alteration in the conscious level during the course of the day from extreme drowsiness to alertness.

A history of head injury is only forthcoming in 50% of patients. When they do remember it is usually mild and occurred within 3 months.

77 The answer is a qualified YES, i.e. whenever possible. Every patient who has had a bump on the head or a lacerated scalp is a potential victim of intracranial haematoma. Two factors are important:

(a) evidence of skull fracture.
(b) evidence of brain damage, e.g. altered conscious level, physical signs etc.

Either of (a) or (b) may occur without the other. Skull fracture can occur without the patient being knocked unconscious. If a fracture is found the patient requires observation for at least 24 hours. It is usually impossible because of resources to admit patients who have neither a fracture nor any signs or symptoms, but who have had a few minutes' amnesia following injury. It is usual to make sure the patient can stay with a responsible friend or relative for observation with the instruction to contact his own doctor or hospital if there is onset of drowsiness, confusion or severe headache.

78 In all cases the diagnosis hangs on the careful history. Examination and investigation rarely reveal abnormal findings. The important features are for example the temporal factors, does it occur at any particular time, in relation to what stimulus, how long does it last etc.

79 (a) Related to emotional circumstances and muscular tension.
(b) Occur mainly in people under 50 years.
(c) Bilateral and often described as being band-like.
(d) Doesn't prevent sleep or cause early wakening.
(e) Usually worse in the evening.
(f) Not relieved by simple analgesics but by tranquillizers.
(g) No abnormal findings on examination.
(h) No change of symptoms over a period of time, i.e. years.

80 There are three areas which must be covered when treating any headache.

(a) Relief of anxiety. Headache is a common symptom known to everyone. Obviously when a patient presents with this symptom, knowing it to be common, the doctor should therefore be alert to the fact that the patient fears a serious underlying cause. The diagnosis should therefore be discussed in such a way as the patient understands the doctor's diagnosis and also is aware that his (the patient's) fears have at least been considered. In some cases it may be necessary to say 'You have nothing at all to worry about because . . .' and go on to explain your negative findings.

Patients with migraine, particularly those who experience focal neurological symptoms, may well fear that they are having a stroke.

(b) Relief of pain. In the case of migraine it is important to relieve the vertigo and vomiting.

(c) Minimize frequency and severity of subsequent attacks.

81 Although the exact mechanism is unknown it appears that the prodromal phase is associated with vascular spasm and the headache and nausea due to vasodilation. It will often respond to large enough doses of simple analgesics if given in the early stages. However, the prodromal symptoms that occur in classical migraine allow us sometimes to abort the subsequent headache and vomiting with ergotamine tartrate.

The earlier ergotamine is given the smaller the required dose will be. Given as nasal snuff it can abort many attacks. Tolerance does not occur but habituation does. It may also be given as suppositories, tablets or by injection. Patients must be careful about dosages as severe side effects occur.

Ergotamine is not a safe prophylactic. Methysergide is the most effective but the serious side effect of retroperitoneal fibrosis can occur with continuous use.

Others worth trying are clonidine, pizotifen and propranolol.

In women who have premenstrual exacerbations then diuretics for 10 days premenstrually can be beneficial.

82   The face of the patient has a characteristic and expressionless appearance. This often alerts the doctor to the diagnosis, as facial movements are slow in starting and tend to be prolonged. Blinking is markedly reduced and tends to occur with the use of voluntary muscles, hence creating the typical appearance known as a 'reptilian gaze'.

The onset of Parkinson's disease is over many months with tremor as a characteristic feature. This usually begins in one limb—often the arm. It spreads to involve the leg on the same side and eventually both sides are affected. It is a rhythmical tremor which disappears on voluntary movement and is of the characteristic 'pill rolling' type. The tremor is aggravated by stress and usually settles during sleep. Rigidity is common in the early stages and resistance to passive movement is increased throughout the whole range of activity of a joint. When the tremor is also present the typical 'cogwheel' resistance is felt.

The patients are usually over the age of 50 and Parkinsonism may be noticed on specific acts such as writing and fine movements. Often the writing is very small and this changes when anti-Parkinsonian treatment is given. Speech can be affected, with slowness and flatness of tone. Rigidity causes a hunchback appearance which, in combination with the hypokinesis, produces the festinant gait. In more advanced cases retropulsion can be disabling.

83   (a) In early cases a discussion of the illness with patient and family is important. The patient must be allowed to discuss his fears for the future. The amount of information imparted must be tempered by the patient's personality and attitude. As time progresses and the condition worsens increasing support will be necessary from the practice team including nurse, health visitor and occupational therapist. Where available, intensive physiotherapy relieves muscle spasm and improves posture.

(b) Anxiety and depression can be prominent features and require treatment with simple tranquillizers and tricyclic antidepressants.

(c) Specific drugs such as L-dopa are best left until the disease is established. They have no effect in halting the disease and only seem to be effective for 2–3 years. After this the frequency of medication is necessarily increased and side effects become prominent.

(d) In the early stages simpler anti-Parkinsonian drugs can be used namely benzhexol and orphenadrine. Amantadine in doses of 100–300 mg daily is often used as an adjuvant but only benefits a proportion of individuals.

(e) The use of bromocriptine remains controversial.

(f) Stereotaxic thalamotomy has now a limited place for the treatment of localized unilateral resting tremor. It seems to have little permanent benefit.

(g) Throughout all drug therapy the patient and family must be supported and national self-help groups are available for information and a newsletter is published.

84 A useful practical general practice test is to ask the patient to see how many words beginning with a particular letter he can produce in one minute. Those with less than ten words probably suffer from dysphasia.

85 The patient may fall to the ground, vomit, sweat profusely and be found lying still with closed eyes and looking pale. When helped up further vomiting occurs and the victim crawls to bed and refuses to move. This may persist for a day or two but the patient gradually adjusts. In the first month any head movement may cause vertigo. The examination reveals severe unidirectional horizontal nystagmus. This nystagmus settles. In the young it accompanies occasionally a viral illness but the cause is unknown. In the elderly it is presumed to be vascular in origin.

The main points are as follows:

(a) Bed rest, reassurance and frequent visiting by either doctor or nurse is beneficial. It is important to stress that they will get better and there is no serious underlying cause.

(b) In the early stages antiemetics like prochlorperazine are helpful and benzodiazapines relieve anxiety.

61

(c) At first injections will be necessary because of nausea and vomiting, but later tablets are adequate.

86 There are two main groups. Those in which the factors are positively correlated (a) and those which are probably correlated (b).

(a) Hypertension—untreated or poorly controlled
Peripheral vascular disease
Raised PCV
Diabetes mellitus
Oral contraceptives
(b) Hyperlipidaemia
Obesity
Lack of exercise
Cigarette smoking

87 There are five areas:

(a) to treat the underlying disease process if this is found to be possible.
(b) to minimize the area of ischaemia and reduce neurosis.
(c) to prevent and treat the complications of acute stroke.
(d) after the event the main thing is to rehabilitate the patient as fully as possible.
(e) to prevent recurrence.

88 Bronchopneumonia is probably the most common sequel to a CVA, particularly in bedfast patients who may also have a bulbar palsy and diminished gag reflex as a result of brain stem involvement. Immobility also can result in deep vein thrombosis in approximately 50% of cases where the lower limbs are paralysed. Many of these are of a subclinical nature. Pulmonary embolism can ocur in about 50% of those dying from CVAs and is the cause of death in some. Of the less serious complications, pressure sores are probably the most common and easily occur even with good nursing care but, naturally, in cases nursed at home the incidence is greater. Urinary infection is common particularly where catheterization has to be carried out. Cardiac rhythm disturbances are common but not often fatal. Contractures can develop in spastic limbs where physiotherapy is not performed. Depression is all too

common in patients with even mild disability at the stage when they come to realize that such a disability is a threat to their normal way of life.

89  There are three main ways:

(a) by increasing intracranial pressure which may manifest as headaches, vomiting and visual disturbance.
(b) by infiltrating normal structures causing loss of function.
(c) by forming a locus for epilepsy.

90  This is a short-lived episode often related to strenuous effort of the previous day. Many of the adolescents which it affects most commonly can remember a forceful action and may even have heard a click. Occasionally it is associated with an acute tonsillitis. The condition is painful, the muscle of one side being in spasm.

The treatment is:

(a) examine for a local cause, i.e. cervical lymphadenopathy.
(b) rest—perhaps in a soft cervical collar.
(c) analgesia—either local with spray or systemic with paracetamol or DF118.
(d) local heat in the form of a partly filled hot water bottle.
(e) benzodiazapine can be useful to relax the very anxious child.

91  This is the commonest mononeuropathy and is due to compression of the median nerve as it passes through the carpal tunnel in the flexor retinaculum. Some of the damage to the nerve is caused by the constant movement of it within the canal with wrist flexion and extension. The tunnel may be narrowed by arthritis in the wrist particularly in patients with rheumatoid arthritis. Occasionally, soft tissue thickening, present in myxoedematous patients can be causative but probably the commonest cause is oedema which occurs normally in pregnancy but is often also a result of drug treatment, e.g. oestrogens. Obesity of a simple nature can be a cause but is less common. Often, however, it is idiopathic. It is more usually found in women and affects the dominant hand first. Patients usually complain of pain and paraesthesiae of the hand and forearm which may wake them at

night but often occurs in the early morning, causing them to get out of bed and shake the hand. Treatment consists of discovering any underlying cause and suitable measures directed towards that cause. In idiopathic cases the most usual first line of treatment is diuretics given in the evening so that any diuresis is over before bedtime. Following this, steroid injections are used, usually of the long acting type, given through the flexor retinaculum. In extreme cases, surgical decompression is indicated.

92 The main point is to establish the causation before treatment is attempted. The main techniques are:

(a) interruption of ascending pain pathways
   (i) peripheral nerve block with local anaesthetic (temporary) or phenol. Local destruction of other modalities may occur.
   (ii) posterior roots—phenol extra, intradurally or subarachnoid. This is usually unselective.
   (iii) spinal chordotomy.
   (iv) brain, thalamotomy and stereotactic procedures.
   (v) pituitary destruction.
(b) techniques to stimulate inhibitory mechanisms
   (i) skin vibration—applied to painful area.
   (ii) electrical stimulation of peripheral nerves. Percutaneous method now much used.
   (iii) acupuncture or electroacupuncture. Especially effective for small bones and joints.
(c) other techniques
   (i) sympathetic block and sympathectomy.
   (ii) biofeedback, relaxation and hypnosis.
   (iii) psychiatric treatment.
   (iv) drugs.

# F Obstetrical problems and gynaecological disorders

93 (a) First of all it is important to understand

what are the individual patient's needs, e.g. does she wish temporary or permanent contraception?

(b) Determine what method she has thought about for herself. (This will often prove to be the best or in any event the most acceptable.)

(c) Take a careful medical history and examine her personal record card to look for contraindications to any particular method, e.g. cardiovascular disease. Check which religious belief she holds.

(d) Explain the advantages and disadvantages of all methods and agree with her the optimum choice.

(e) Prescribe the method of choice and ensure she understands how it should be used (or taken).

(f) Arrange follow-up.

94 (a) Describe how the pill works and exactly what it is.

(b) Counting the first day of the period as day one then she should take the first pill on day five, whether the period has finished or not. It is better to use additional precautions for the first 14 days of the first cycle.

(c) It is important to take the pill at approximately the same time each day.

(d) When the packet is finished then the period usually starts 2 or 3 days later. Take the first pill of the next packet on 7th day after finishing the previous packet, i.e. if she finished the first pack on a Tuesday she is to start the second pack the following Tuesday.

(e) If she has the pill she is likely to experience shorter, lighter periods. Also mention the possible side effects of the pill and the warning signs. Explain the significance of breakthrough bleeding and that she needs to see her GP if it occurs more than once.

(f) If she suffers an attack of diarrhoea or vomiting of more than a day then she is to continue the pill, but she should take additional precautions for the remainder of the cycle.

95 It is now normal to commence oral contaception 4 weeks after delivery, since ovulation has

not commenced. There is no need to await menstruation as used to be believed. This was so as not to miss Sheehan's syndrome presenting as amenorrhoea but since this is much less common as a result of better third stage control there is no need to await the first period.

In breast feeding mothers this very act serves as a partial contraceptive but it is unreliable as a method and some advice should be given. It is also normal for breast feeding mothers to have amenorrhoea which returns to normal when the child is weaned. The combined pill is not the method of choice in these cases as the flow of breast milk tends to stop. The progestogen-only pill is a useful alternative and the combined pill can be started (if mother so wishes) when the breast feeding is terminated.

96 (a) Superficial thrombosis. This is much commoner in pill users with varicose veins. It is also related to the strength of the pill and it is obviously better that women should be taking the weakest but effective pill which suits them. Superficial thrombosis is 2–5 times more common in pill takers than non-users.
   (b) Deep vein thrombosis. This is not related to the presence of varicose veins, but to the total dose of the pill or its individual components. This complication is 4 times commoner in women on the combined pill.
   (c) Hypertension. This is usually reversible, but can occur in 5% of users after 5 years.
   (d) Circulatory disease. The incidence of heart disease is related to age and cigarette smoking. It is very much increased in cigarette smokers over 35 years of age and it is in this group that alternative methods are prescribed.

97 (a) Prescribe a pill with lower oestrogen content.
   (b) First of all prescribe a pill with a higher progestogen content, but if this fails then use a pill with high oestrogen dose plus progestogen content.
   (c) Stop the pill.
   (d) Increase progestogen dose.

98    (a) Anti-infective agents, e.g. rifampicin, ampicillin, sulphamethoxypyridazine.

    (b) Barbiturates, e.g. hexobarbitone and phenobarbitone.

    (c) Vasoconstrictors e.g. ergot compounds.

    (d) Tranquillizers, e.g. chlorpromazine, chlordiazepoxide and meprobamate.

    (e) Anticonvulsants e.g. phenytoin, primidone, ethosuximide.

99    In those patients who are forgetful and are irritated by, or tend to omit regular procedures, IUCDs are obviously an advantage. They are also advantageous in those patients who have significant worries about hormonal contraception and in whom hormones are contraindicated. In addition, mothers who are breast feeding suffer no impairment of that facility when fitted with an IUCD. After insertion and apart from regular checking by the patients themselves, there is no need to replenish supplies and it cannot be left behind when going on holiday. Once inserted, definite action is needed to counteract the contraceptive effect. Regarding effectiveness, it is second only to the combined pill and has a lower incidence of serious side effects.

100    It affects up to 30% of women during the reproductive phase of their lives. Some women date the onset to having become pregnant. In others it may occur soon after puberty. Yet a third group notice symptoms only in the few years prior to the menopause. It is characterized by agitation, depression, irritability and bad temper during the few days prior to the onset of menstruation. No-one can be sure of the causation. Some workers suggest that the basic cause is oestrogen/progestogen imbalance and measurement of blood levels in such cases are, indeed, high. These levels affect the status of other hormones and it is felt that this interdependence is the cause of the varied nature of the syndrome. Because of the widespread nature of this complaint, it is important to exclude true endogeneous depression as this can also have premenstrual excerbations.

101    (a) Reassurance and explanation. Diuretics for 7 days prior to menstruation often help when weight gain is a prominent feature.

(b) Vitamin B—pyridoxine 50 mg daily. This is helpful in up to 50% of patients.

(c) Progesterone orally in the 2nd half of the cycle, the commonest one used in practice being dydrogesterone.

(d) The combined oral contraceptive is often helpful but usually a high dosage pill must be used continuously.

(e) Danazol to suppress gonadotrophin production. This is only helpful if ovarian function is overcome.

102 (a) Chronic pelvic inflammatory disease. Here the long history will give the diagnosis when previously intercourse was pain free. Promiscuity and tuberculous contacts are pointers also. Appropriate antibiotic therapy is usually curative, although local surgical removal may be indicated.

(b) Endometriosis. This may require laparoscopy for assessment. Danazol usually settles the symptoms.

(c) Uterine retroversion. The dyspareunia is usually due to discomfort caused by low lying ovaries. Here a change of coital position can help, although surgical correction is often needed.

(d) Vault discomfort may follow hysterectomy, ventrosuspension or irradiation. Change of coital position is helpful.

103 Frankly, at present, the treatment of the herpes II virus lesions is very unsatisfactory.

In some women the pain is agonizing and passing urine is extremely painful and even catheterization has been performed. One useful ploy is to suggest passing urine while bathing, but this recommendation may offend some individuals.

The application of saline packs is comforting and systemic conventional analgesics can be prescribed.

The early use of idoxuridine 0.5% in dimethylsulphoxide may abort in some cases and this is available as an ointment to be applied 2-hourly.

A new preparation, acyclovir, is now available both for oral administration and as a cream. It appears to be effective in a high proportion of cases. The oral dose is 200 mg 5 times daily for 5 days which may need to be extended in patients with severe infection. The cream needs to be applied with the same frequency.

104 Probably the commonest single cause now is moniliasis. This can be confirmed by swab and sent on a slide or in transport medium to the laboratory. In the past the only treatments were local, using cream and/or cut-up pessaries inserted by mother plus oral nystatin to sterilize the gut, the major drawback, of course, being the need to 'interfere' with the child. Ketoconazole, 100 g twice daily for 5 days is now the treatment of choice. If there is no response to treatment then the possibility of an inserted foreign body must be considered. This may be easily removable but often can only be suspected. In these cases examination under GA is mandatory.

105 (a) Oral contraceptive usage.
(b) The use of broad spectrum antibiotics which kill protective organisms.
(c) Diabetes mellitus.
(d) Pregnancy.

106 *Age of beginning smears*. All women in any group who wish a smear should be offered one but the high risk groups are girls under 20 years with a history of termination of pregnancy, promiscuity or veneral disease. Those seen for contraceptive advice at this age should also have a smear. In the remainder 22 years is the common age to start taking smears especially in those who are pregnant.

*Frequency*. A second smear should be taken a year after the first so as to guard against false negatives. After this 3-yearly is the optimum rate if the patient is over 35 years or 4-yearly if under 35 years of age.

*Age of cessation*. It is usual to stop at 70 years.

107 A full gynaecological history is naturally helpful, but there is need to concentrate on what symptoms are causing most trouble. There are three major groups of symptoms.

(a) The first is due to lack of oestradiol and caused by the involution of the tissues which depend on a supply of oestradiol for nutrition, e.g. atrophy of breast and lower genital tract.

(b) Second are due to overstimulation by pituitary hormones affecting changes in the vasomotor system. This results in attacks of flushing and sweating which can be debilitating and are a cause of insomnia.

(c) Third are the psychological and psychiatric symptoms which can occur, particularly in susceptible women. The menopause occurs at a time of life when the children are leaving home, when social and work commitments can be at their greatest and when the husband is at his maximum earning potential. With the atrophy of their sexual characteristics, some women fear a loss of sexual appeal and feel their femininity is waning. Conversely some women feel guilty that their sexual drive is not diminishing and that it ought to in proportion to their loss of physical sexual attraction. It is vital to allow the patient to air her feelings and discuss her symptoms and fears. This on its own may allow her to struggle through. The general practitioner should discuss the range of normality to see where she fits in the scale. Medical treatment is then the result of discussion and by mutual agreement.

108 (a) Hormone replacement therapy is still a controversial subject and its introduction is a time for full discussion with the patient. Carefully selected patients, however, have a dramatic reversal of symptoms. It is essential that treatment should commence with low doses and that the minimum dose consistent with alleviation of symptoms be used. Treatment should be given cyclically for 3 weeks out of 4. Most phased treatments involve the use of oestrogens and progestogens in a changing combination during the cycle of administration.

(b) Vasomotor symptoms when occurring alone or when they are the prominent feature may be treated with chemicals which restrict vasomotor response. The most common of these is clonidine.

(c) The psychological and psychiatric symptoms may require specific psychotropic drugs but often discussion and reassurance is sufficient. Agitation and insomnia may

70

be relieved by simple minor tranquillizers such as the benzodiazepines, but it is important to exclude major psychiatric illness which may present with agitation. It is useful to stress the temporary nature of the climacteric and to give continuing support to vulnerable individuals.

109 (a) Ensure that the patient is in fact pregnant and less than 16 weeks' gestation.
(b) Check the history of contact and the validity of the diagnosis.
(c) Has the patient clinical rubella?
(d) Check rubella antibody titres. If the patient has children already then it is probable that the immunity state has been verified and the vaccine given if she had been susceptible. If this is her first pregnancy she may have been immune at the outset because of childhood infection or immunization. If the patient is susceptible then a rising antibody titre after 2 weeks indicates infection. If this infection has taken place in the first 8 weeks of pregnancy then there is a 60% chance that the child will be affected to some degree. These risks must be discussed with the patient and termination offered. There is no evidence that gammaglobulin is protective. The risks to the fetus decrease progressively after 8 weeks' gestation and are negligible after 16 weeks.

110 If possible *all* drugs in early pregnancy should be avoided. The most liable to produce problems are:

(a) cytotoxic agents—the worst being folic acid antagonists and alkylating agents.
(b) all the drugs used to control epilepsy have been implicated.
(c) alcohol
(d) lithium
(e) quinine
(f) warfarin
(g) co-trimoxazole (Septrin)

It must be emphasized however that some of the above risks are theoretical only.

111 *Advantages*
   (a) Mother is the centre of the occasion in her own territory and is in charge of the process.
   (b) She is free to conduct herself in the first stage of labour as she wishes, e.g. position, ambulation, food etc. It is important to be mobile in the first stage to make labour progress normally.
   (c) Lower anxiety level in mother because she doesn't have to worry about the timing of leaving for hospital. She is in her own surroundings. Provided the mother is relaxed then labour progresses normally.
   (d) The attitude to birth is accepting, supportive and exciting. This aids bonding.
   (e) Because of (a) to (d) less sedation and analgesia is usually required, there are thus benefits to the fetus/baby.
   (f) Cross-infection is much less a problem.
   (g) Breast feeding more easily established.
   (h) Integration with the rest of the family is usually easier because of involvement.

   *Disadvantages*
   (a) Poor back-up facilities for ante and post partum haemorrhage premature and precipitate labour. Inadequate resuscitation available.
   (b) No fetal and maternal monitoring facilities.
   (c) Greater load on mother and family during and after delivery.
   (d) Present midwifery and medical staff are poorly trained to handle home confinements.
   (e) Anxiety in mother as to what may happen if an emergency arises.

112 (a) She may claim she has a poor milk supply. This is usually because she is unconvinced about the benefits of breast feeding. It is psychogenic in origin in most cases.
   (b) Social life inhibited. Because of the usual 3-hourly regimen and the fact that her presence is naturally vital then she is severely limited in how much social life she can have outside of the home.
   (c) Husband objects to breast feeding. Occasionally husbands do feel jealous about the amount of attention the child receives and the fact that he cannot join in.

(d) Baby irritable. This is usually because mother is unable to relax and allow the let-down reflex to take place. This diminishes the milk supply.

(e) Social embarrassment. Many mothers feel completely unable to feed their children except in the comfort and seculsion of their own home. This tends to be a Western habit.

(f) Painful nipples. This is often due to the baby getting an inadequate milk supply and demanding more.

(g) It may be that she has stopped on medical advice, e.g. she has had to start on medication which passes into the breast milk. Also if factors (a), (d) or (f) have been discussed with her doctor it is likely that breast feeding will need to be discontinued for the benefit of both mother and child.


## G  Disorders of ear, nose and throat

113 It is difficult to be certain here because authorities differ in their exact incidence and prevalences but the good average would be 15%. In other words approximately every sixth patient is presenting with an ENT problem.

There is of course a seasonal and social class variation.

114 The vast majority of acute and chronic ear problems in childhood are due to the blocking of the eustachian tube. The major causes of this are as follows.

(a) Hereditary—much ear disease tends to run in families and an inherited tendency to narrow or angular eustachian tubes means that there is a predisposition to blocking.

(b) Upper respiratory infection. Viral damage to lining cells causes oedema and tube blockage. This is the commonest factor.

(c) Adenoidal enlargement. Hypertrophy can involve tissue near eustachian tube entrances and oedema can block off drainage.

(d) Rhinitis—this may be allergic or non-specific but often involves the tube with consequent failure of pressure equalization.

115 First of all the diagnosis must be confirmed by otoscope and to some extent the management depends on the previous history and the social circumstances.

Viral causes account for about 70% of cases but recurrent attacks with previous perforations demand early antibiotic therapy. Children in families below social class three will probably require antibiotics because mothers are less likely to bring them for follow-up and audiometry.

The most likely organisms when bacterial are:

(a) *Haemophilus influenzae*—especially in the under-fives.
(b) Pneumococci.
(c) *Streptococcus pyogenes*.

A reasonable course of management would be:

acute earache
↓
give analgesics (soluble aspirin etc.)

give antibiotics to social classes 4 and 5 and those with previous pathology ↓ review 3 weeks for follow-up and arrange audiometry ↓ interim follow-up by health visitor to ensure medication being taken

review 2 days

not settled ↓ use amoxycillin for under-fives; use penicillin V or cotrimoxazole for over-fives ↓ review 3 weeks and arrange audiometry in 3 months

settled or settling, review 3 weeks

116 Wax in the auditory canal is by far the commonest diagnosis. Wax may be removed by one of two methods:

(a) by forceps or suction
(b) by syringing

Removal by forceps or suction must usually be carried out in the hospital and this will necessitate referral. Which of the two methods is appropriate will, to a large extent, depend on the past history. If previous suction has been performed then there was obviously a good reason for it. It is important to examine the past history carefully for evidence of chronic suppurative otitis media or previous perforation.

If the drum is intact and there is not previous significant history it is possible to syringe the external auditory canal. The principles are:

(a) Soften the wax as much as possible by the patient using olive or almond oil for 5 days prior to the procedure.
(b) Protect the patient from water overflow.
(c) Check water temperature and make sure it is at body temperature, as discrepancies can cause vertigo.
(d) Gently but firmly direct a jet of water at the ceiling of the external auditory canal at the same time gently withdrawing the pinna upwards and backwards. Collect the used water and wax in a tank held by the patient under the appropriate ear.
(e) Check the canal and drum afterwards for any underlying pathology.

A hitherto previously unknown perforation will be discovered by the patient commenting that he can feel water trickling down the back of his throat. If this is noticed, stop the procedure immediately, note the fact in the patient's record and administer suitable antibiotics. The drug of first choice is Septrin

117 Obviously it should be removed, but it depends on two variables:

(a) the child
(b) the foreign body

If the child is very young or distressed it is often necessary to remove foreign bodies under general anaesthesia. Most children cooperate well if handled sympathetically and with reasonable explanations given. Sometimes it is easier if the parent is present, but the converse can often apply. The two major methods are using:

(a) water, by syringe—the jet blows out the foreign body and it works particularly well for insects and floating objects such as beads.
(b) forceps—useful for irregular objects or when the foreign body completely blocks the canal. The other rarer indication is when the object is organic and could

possibly swell when in contact with water, e.g. dried peas.

118 Four to six months is the earliest feasible opportunity for hearing tests to be carried out.

Usually the child is visited in his home environment, although in some areas children are brought to a central point. Obviously home testing has a lot of advantages mainly because of the relaxed nature of the child. The tests are carried out by an experienced health visitor.

The baby tends to turn his head in the direction from which the sound is coming and this is best done with the sounds at ear level and preferably made by familiar objects. The objects should be chosen so as to check different frequency ranges:

(a) spoon in feeding cup.
(b) mother's voice calling his name.
(c) rattle (favourite)—also high and low pitch.
(d) rustling paper.
(e) ringing of bells.
(f) hissing.

After 9 months of age a variety of sounds may be used which can be fed through an amplifier.

As the child grows older then a command game can be instituted. The basis of this is that the child performs a task in response to a command it hears. The sound stimulus meanwhile varies in pitch and intensity and is measured on a metre.

A pure tone audiogram cannot be done under 4 years of age.

119 This tends to be a recurring problem and it is important to help the patient understand this. Since the skin lining the auditory canal is in many ways like ordinary skin it may react to a generalized skin disorder.

(a) Swab the discharge from the ear—this may not, however, be helpful as a mixed colony growth is typical.
(b) In the acute phase insert a glycerine and icthammol wick. This should be done only in one ear at a time as it renders the

patient totally deaf. This preparation is
hygroscopic and analgesic.
(c) In the less acute phase use a combined
antibiotic/steroid ointment either directly
inserted in the ear or absorbed onto a wick.

Frequent dressing may be necessary and
aural toilet prior to re-instilling ointment is
beneficial always providing the patient can
bear the discomfort. Here lies the dilemma
because the more pain the patient experiences
tends to be proportional to the extent to which
aural toilet is necessary.

120 There is a large psychosomatic component to
this illness and a sympathetic and understanding approach is necessary. It is useful to explain
carefully the nature and cause of the illness and
involve the patient in discussion of the management.
The various medical possibilities include:

(a) restriction of salt intake.
(b) labyrinth sedatives such as betahistine.
(c) vasodilators.
(d) tranquillizers.
(e) anti-smoking advice.

If these measures do not control the problem
then the vestibular mechanism can be des-
troyed by ultrasound. In other centres alternative surgical treatments include vestibular
neurectomy or decompression of the saccus
endolymphaticus.

121 By far the commonest cause is positional vertigo which accounts for at least 80% of the
cases presenting to a GP. On average a GP can
expect to see about 7 cases per annum.
The second commonest cause is Menière's
disease which accounts for about 15% of cases.
The remainder of cases are made up of acute
infective episodes, chronic otitis media, transient ischaemic attacks and the acute manifestations of demyelinating diseases.

122 (a) Acute onset of sensation of rotation on
head movement associated with nausea
and vomiting.

(b) Vertigo much worse with head movement. Usually the easiest position is lying flat.

(c) Nystagmus is usually present but other physical signs are lacking.

(d) Attacks tend to affect young or middle aged adults and pass off spontaneously in a few days. Recurrent attacks can occur however.

123 Bearing in mind that the commonest causes are positional vertigo and Menière's syndrome it is important to take a full history and a selective neurological examination. The important elements to check are:

(a) fundi—exclude raised intracranial pressure, multiple sclerosis etc.

(b) BP, pulse and apex beat (to exclude emboli, hypertension etc.).

(c) tendon reflexes—to exclude CVA.

(d) examine for hearing loss—Menière's syndrome.

It is important to reassure the patient and the family that the condition is not serious and that you have excluded stroke, hypertension, and cerebral tumour as causes.

Acquaint the patient and family of the natural course of the illness and that it will settle in a few days.

Give general advice about the illness namely: to rest flat as much as possible until symptoms settle and to reduce head movements to a minimum. Ambulation should only be as rapid as recovery allows. Driving should be forbidden temporarily.

Symptomatic relief is often afforded with prochlorperazine or promethazine.

Review and careful follow-up should be carried out.

124 When long term exposure has taken place to continuous loud noise then sensorineural deafness occurs. It is typically high tone loss and a classical audiogram will show a dip at 4000 Hz.

Usually the worker will admit to not wearing hearing protectors when questioned closely.

125 The most effective method is the fitting of one and sometimes two maskers. These are small devices rather like hearing aids which emit a masking sound but don't obstruct the meatus.

The low level white sound suppresses the much louder tinnitus of a different frequency spectrum. Approximately two-thirds of such patients can be helped.

126   (a) Viral pharyngitis. Sore throat occurs in conjunction with fever, headaches, tonsillar enlargement and often creamy white exudates. In many cases the cervical nodes are enlarged. The commonest implicated viruses are adenoviruses and coxsackie viruses.

(b) Streptococcal sore throat. The appearances can be identical to the above and clinically it is just not possible to separate the causes on clinical grounds. A throat swab can be helpful in this. There is a great deal of debate as to whether penicillin or erythromycin should be used 'blindly'. The protagonists say that these are cheap antibiotics which rarely do any harm, but can be very helpful. The subscribers to the non-antibiotic regimen say there is good objective evidence that whether antibiotics are used or not, the time taken to recover is the same and that such wanton prescribing reinforces the need for patients to return on future infective occasions.

(c) Infectious mononucleosis. Here, in addition to the above symptoms, there may be splenomegaly and even hepatomegaly. Also a faint skin rash may be present plus petechiae on the soft palate. The Epstein–Barr virus is causative and an allergic rash in response to ampicillin therapy is almost always present if this drug is used.

127   The three major indications are:

(a) any individual who suffers from tonsillitis with 'toxic' symptoms (dysphagia, fever, malaise) on more than three occasions in a year.

(b) having had a peritonsillar abscess.

(c) recurrent pyrexial fits.

128   In children the bleeding site tends to be Little's area. A calm reassuring approach is essential as this is an alarming occurrence for youngsters.

(a) Sit the child upright with the nose dripping into a basin.

(b) Get the patient to blow his nose into the basin and decide which nostril is bleeding.

(c) If available insert cotton wool half soaked in 4% lignocaine and adrenaline hydrochloride 1:1000 solution and tell the child or persuade mother to pinch the nostril so the cotton wool is in contact with Little's area. If no solution is available then place an ice cube on either side of the nose and likewise pinch for 10 minutes.

(d) When bleeding is arrested cauterize the bleeding points either chemically or electrically if found.

In the elderly the bleeding point is usually high and out of sight. In many cases hypertension is the underlying cause.

(a) Prop the patient up as above.

(b) Spray inside both nostrils with 4% lignocaine and 1:1000 adrenaline.

(c) Either pack both nostrils with gauze soaked in the above solution or insert inflatable balloon packs. It is feasible to use urinary balloon cathethers (30 ml) for this purpose.

(d) Check general condition of cardiovascular system and patient's general state.

(e) Arrange care either at home or admission to hospital.

(f) Remove pack after 48 hours.

129  First of all it is essential to try and establish what the underlying causes may be.

(a) Excessive alcohol consumption—usually there are other indicators of value, e.g. MCV, gamma glutamyl transferase, history from spouse.

(b) Excessive smoking—this may be the whole problem or merely a contributing factor.

(c) Direct irritants—these may be at work or in the home.

(d) Hypersensitivity—often to pollens, house dust etc. In these cases skin testing may be valuable but the majority of individuals with an allergic response tend to react to several similar allergens. Desensitization is less popular than formerly and should only be done where full resuscitation measures are available.

(e) Psychogenic. It is important to check that the sinuses are clear and radiology is helpful here. The mainstay of therapy is supportive. It is essential to avoid any allergen as much as possible. Desensitization is really only useful for single allergens.

The next stage is the intermittent use of antihistamines and topical steroid sprays. Occasionally systemic steroids may be necessary, e.g. at the height of the pollen season. In resistant cases submucosal diathermy is helpful.

130 In the younger age group, i.e. under 40 years, then after giving advice on non-smoking and alcohol reduction it is reasonable to wait a period of 3 weeks after the onset of symptoms before referral for direct laryngoscopy.

With the over 40 age group you should suspect laryngeal carcinoma until proven otherwise when 2 weeks have elapsed from the onset of symptoms.

During the waiting period additional counselling regarding voice rest should be given.

131 In many cases pain around the ear and behind it is common and may precede the paralysis by up to 2 days. The onset of facial weakness may be reported as sudden but it may also gradually progress over a course of up to 4 days. There may be spontaneous complaint of loss of taste, watering of the eye and increased sensitivity to sound on the side affected. There may also be transient numbness of the affected side of the face or of the tongue. This may be due to trigeminal nerve involvement but it is probably an unpleasant awareness of the paralysis. The severity of the facial weakness varies from slight to complete but all the muscles of the face are always affected to some degree. In the elderly, facial distortion is much more pronounced and drooping of the lower lid is obvious. The face may appear to be drawn up on the normal side and this may be the complaint of the patient who believes that it is the normal side which is affected.

## H  Disorders of the circulatory system

132    The diagnosis rests almost entirely on the history. Classically angina occurs on exertion and it is difficult, therefore, to examine the patient when the pain is present. Usually the pain passes quickly on resting. It is exacerbated by cold weather and often occurs after meals. There is often a central chest discomfort (described as someone sitting on the chest), with heaviness and tightness radiating to the left arm and often the jaw. Occasionally epigastric pain is described. Dyspnoea is also common. It can occur in relation to stress and emotion and can occasionally occur at night (the so-called Prinzmetal syndrome).

133    (a) The typical crushing pain may not present on effort, but when the cardiovascular system is stretched by other demands, e.g. for digestion after a meal, in cold weather, or by excitement inducing tachycardia.
       (b) The pain may not occur across the chest on exertion, e.g. in the jaw or upper abdomen. It is the relationship to exercise which gives it away in this case.
       (c) It is possible that breathlessness is the prominent symptom rather than chest pain or perhaps extreme breathlessness associated with a little chest discomfort.

134    There are two basic principles namely eating the correct amount of the correct foods.

       (a) A target weight relating to age and sex should be given and supervision organized to help the patient accomplish this.
       (b) Correct eating consists of:

           (i) eating less meat and few egg yolks and cheese, grilled food in preference to fried, avoiding fat and eating more poultry and fish.
           (ii) avoiding butter and using polyunsaturated margarine; foregoing cream and top of the milk.
           (iii) using polyunsaturated oils in cooking.

135    (a) Stopping smoking; improves both prognosis and symptoms.
       (b) Sublingual glyceryl trinitrate; for relief

during attacks and as a prophylactic prior
to exertion.

(c) Beta-blockers; acting on beta-adrenergic
receptors, reduce heart rate and blood
pressure. In some cases there is also a
central action. They may also limit the
degree of damage if infarction occurs.

(d) Long acting nitrates; such as isosorbide.

(e) Calcium antagonists; such as nifedipine
and verapamil.

(f) Referral for assessment regarding cardiac
surgery.

136 (a) The tablet should be dissolved slowly
under the tongue. If they are swallowed
then absorption is slower and most of the
drug is metabolized in the liver and doesn't
reach the heart.

(b) If the pain is severe the tablet can be
crunched and the pieces allowed to dis-
solve under the tongue.

(c) The episodes of activity which produce
pain which can be anticipated should be
preceded by using a tablet.

(d) Several small bottles of tablets should be
distributed throughout different clothes so
the patient is never without tablets.

(e) Since the active ingredient evaporates then
small tightly stoppered bottles should be
used and the tablets replaced every 6 or 9
months.

(f) In some people a pounding headache is
produced and this should be worried about
but this is normal and not a side effect.
It can be reduced by using a half tablet or
spitting out the remainder when the pain is
eased.

(g) Explain that TNT is not addictive and as
many as are necessary can be used. The
effect does not diminish with use.

(h) There are no drug interactions of any con-
sequence.

(i) Angina should be relieved in a few minutes
and if present after 30 minutes then a
doctor should be consulted.

137 The mortality rate for acute myocardial infarction is approximately 50%. Of these, in the first
hour approximately 35% of patients die and a
further 10% die in the second hour. This means

that of myocardial deaths then approximately half occur in the first 2 hours and in the vast majority of cases the patient has not, by that time, reached the intensive care unit.

Unless a pain is dramatic or severe a patient is unlikely to call his GP immediately. Commonly an hour has elapsed from the onset of pain, to the point when the GP arrives. It is important for the patient to be stabilized before transfer to a coronary unit and continuous observation should be carried out during the move. This may mean bringing the coronary team to the patient's home.

138   In most cases the bradycardia is due to para-sympathetic overactivity. If the patient is normotensive then there is no need to treat this finding and the pulse rate will gradually come back to normal with analgesia.

If the patient is hypertensive then the outlook is much more serious and transfer to a CCU is advisable after giving atropine 0.6 mg IV slowly.

139   Usually the shortness of breath is due to heart failure causing back pressure on the lung. Why should this suddenly occur? Often the infarction has involved one of the papillary muscles which supports the valves. This muscle then softens and ruptures and causes the valve to become incompetent, hence leading to failure.

140   (a) The original role is in the diagnosis of angina.

(b) The submaximal exercise test can be used even 8 days after an uncomplicated myocardial infarction. Pronounced ST interval depression predicts sudden cardiac death within the first year post-infarction. This correlates well with coronary angiography. The pattern on the ECG indicates which arteries are involved by atheroma. This allows early referral for assessment and surgery.

(c) During the rehabilitation stage it demonstrates to the patient how much exercise he is capable of and is reasurring to him and his family.

141   Most ordinary work is not resumed until 2–3

months after a myocardial infarction. Intercourse is a mixed isometric and isotonic exercise with wide variations in heart rate and blood pressure. There is a substantial increase in cardiac work which can be limited to some extent by beta-blockers. The main benefits of early resumption (within 4 weeks of the event) is that it avoids invalidism, sexual difficulties, depression and excessive drug usage.

142   The two main ways are:

(a) screening
(b) case finding.

*Screening.* Here all patients within a chosen age group are sent for and checked by either doctor or nurse. There are bound to be defaulters, but a system for finding these can be defined and if a second letter fails to produce results then a home visit is necessary.

*Case finding.* This system depends on the patient attending the surgery for some unrelated reason, e.g. sore throat, coil check and having their BP taken routinely. Eighty per cent of patients visit their doctor within 3 years and 95 per cent visit within 5 years. What is vital is good record keeping so a recorded BP is easily seen. Also a foolproof system of follow-up is essential.

It is then a relatively small task to send for the remainder of patients who have not recently seen the doctor and they can be 'screened'.

143   (a) That the patient should remain symptom free.
(b) To minimize drug side effects.
(c) To lower both systolic and diastolic blood pressures within the satifactory range.
(d) Whenever possible to keep treatment regimens simple and drug costs to a minimum.
(e) To allow the patient to maintain a satisfactory life style which will increase treatment compliance.

144   (a) Patient education. It is important that each patient understands what hypertension is and what are the implications of poor

control. It is important to actively involve the patient in the management of his disease.

(b) Patient support. Since medication and supervision is likely to be life long then all possible support should be given. This may include introduction of self-help groups.

(c) Abolition of cigarette smoking.

(d) Weight reduction and dieting counselling.

(e) Reduction of other risk factors which includes increasing exercise, controlling diabetes mellitus.

(f) Stopping oral contraceptives and recommending other forms of contraception and stopping other aggravating chemicals, e.g. alcohol in excess, liquorice and carbenoxolone.

(g) Patients should be advised to reduce their salt intake to 6 g/day.

(h) The introduction of relaxation therapy, yoga and biofeedback have been shown to be useful.

145  (a) Machine problems.
    (i) Stuck and dirty valves.
    (ii) Dirty mercury column.
    (iii) Tight clothing above cuff.
    (iv) Cuff applied too loosely, balloon not over radial artery or cuff simply too small.

   (b) Doctor error
    (i) Mercury column allowed to fall too quickly—auscultatory gap.
    (ii) Phase IV or V reading. (Most investigators now use phase V.)
    (iii) Terminal digit preference.
    (iv) Doctor's attitude to hypertension.

   (c) Patient error
    (i) Posture—sitting, lying or standing.
    (ii) Diurnal variation.
    (iii) Values become lower over subsequent visits.
    (iv) Degree of obesity.

146  The use of diuretics. They are at their most effective in treating chronic left-sided congestive failure but relatively unhelpful in the primarily right-sided variety. Management consists of balancing cardiac output against the reduction of end-diastolic pressure. Intravenous diuretics can dramatically reduce the

end-diastolic pressure and remove pulmonary oedema.

Usually with modern drugs an adequate effect can be achieved and when under control the drug dosage needs to be reduced since continuing with unnecessarily high dosages reduces cardiac output. This produces symptoms of fatigue, lethargy and a rising blood urea.

147  (a) Change to a potassium sparing diuretic such as spironolactone or amiloride.
 (b) An orange or a grapefruit taken daily are equivalent to slow release potassium preparations and are much more acceptable.

It is advisable to check serum potassium about 4–6 weeks after commencing diuretic therapy as most hypokalaemics present early. An annual check thereafter is adequate but obviously indicated in any patient complaining of fatigue while taking loop diuretics.

In patients who require large doses of loop diuretics such as frusemide, the addition of potassium sparing preparations not only limits potassium loss but also increases the diuretic effect.

148  (a) Immobility particularly in association with surgery or after trauma or when infection is present or IV cannulae *in situ*.
 (b) Patients who have had previous thrombotic disease or have a genetic tendency.
 (c) Pregnancy in those on the combined oral contraceptive pill. The risks increase with age.
 (d) After myocardial infarction.
 (e) With increasing age.
 (f) Malignancy, particularly pancreatic.
 (g) The presence of varicose veins.
 (h) Obesity.

149  Because the blood flow is impaired then any increase which may be desirable is not possible. The healing ability of old tissues is therefore reduced and trauma should be avoided at all costs. If infection is allowed to occur then severe impairment can result with frank gangrene taking place. Since the normal barriers to infection are hampered then normally benign

bacteria can prove difficult to treat, e.g. *Staphylococcus albus*. It is essential that the patient has professional chiropody.

The inability to respond by vasodilatation means that heat applied to the ischaemic skin cannot be conducted away and burns easily occur. The patient should be told to wash the limb in lukewarm or cold water only.

In order to prevent vasoconstriction of the limb in cold weather the patient must wrap up warmly throughout his body.

150 All the methods below are designed to increase vascular flow.

(a) Elevation of the bed-head. This increases gravitational effect and improves the circulation to the limbs.
(b) Alcohol, taken as a nightcap can cause sufficient vasodilatation as to abolish the pain.
(c) Quinine bisulphate in a dose of 300 mg acts directly on vascular smooth muscle. Some patients have a 'cure' after only 4 weeks' therapy but others require continuous medication.

# I  Disorders of the respiratory system

151 Given a practice population of 2400 patients in an average town approximately 25% of workload will be due to respiratory illness. The vast majority of these are mild and self-limiting conditions, but approximately 40% of sickness is due to respiratory illness.

In any one year he is likely to see approximately:

| | |
|---|---|
| Colds | 180–200 cases |
| Lobar pneumonia | 10 cases |
| Acute bronchitis | 200 cases |
| Cough | 300 cases |
| Chronic bronchitis | 20 cases |
| Influenza | 30 cases |
| Allergic asthma | 20 cases |
| Bronchogenic carcinoma | 2 or 3 cases |

152 Most smokers wish to give up smoking and GP advice still has the greatest success rate. Be-

tween 9% and 5% permanently stop smoking with GP's help.

(a) Careful smoking history should be taken, e.g. association with tension situations etc.
(b) Advise regarding reduction of consumption at first to one cigarette after meals and light the first cigarette 10 minutes later each day.
(c) List the adverse effects on general health, e.g. reduced exercise tolerance, reduced resistance to infection. Point out the diseases in which smoking is positively correlated namely acute and chronic bronchitis; carcinoma of larynx, lung, oesophagus and stomach; peptic ulceration; hypertension; ischaemic heart disease; and peripheral vascular disease. Mention the effects on family and children. Fetal growth is retarded. When young a child in a smoker's house suffers more from respiratory illness. The subsequent effect is that these children are more likely to smoke. Overall is the cost.
(d) Encouragement to stop should be positive. Specially advantageous opportunities are at routine medicals, antenatal clinics, child care clinics and special observation clinics, e.g. diabetics and hypertensives.
   If the patient develops a smoking-related disease the opportunity to give advice should not be missed.
(e) Back-up leaflets should be given, e.g. 'Give up smoking' available from the Health Education Council.
(f) Use 'Nicorette' chewing gum in suitable patients. There are two strengths, 2 mg and 4 mg. The rate of chewing affects absorption and it is especially helpful in heavy smokers in maintaining nicotine levels while they are coping with the social and psychological effects of stopping.
(g) Follow-up whenever possible and record progress in the notes. It is disheartening for patients to attempt to give up and their doctor not be interested in their progress.

153 There is very little published evidence to support the theory that certain families are resistant to the effect of cigarette smoking. Conversely, however, those individuals with an

αantitrypsin deficiency are very much more susceptible to the harmful effects of smoking.

In the general population the dangers are dose related.

154 This is the most common respiratory symptom and is present in 60% of respiratory illness presenting to general practitioners. Their reasons for seeking advice are:

(a) fear that an upper respiratory infection has spread 'down onto the chest'.
(b) insomnia—there is increased stress in families in small houses or where there is shared accommodation. It is common for fathers kept awake to insist that mother takes the child to his GP the next day because of inability to sleep.
(c) fear of carcinoma of the bronchus, asthma or tuberculosis. It is important to discuss these possibilities in the consultation and to show the patient or relative that you understand their anxiety and that your arrangement plan is realistic in their circumstances.

155 (a) Prescribed therapy will need to be taken during the pollen season (predominantly May–August) and the side effects must be explained. The major precaution is to warn antihistamine takers about associated drowsiness and particularly when driving and operating machinery.
(b) Avoid high pollen concentration when possible. Pollen count is highest on humid warm days after rain and particularly if it is windy. Particularly troublesome is a car or train journey with an open window. House windows should be kept shut whenever possible.
(c) Do not go camping.
(d) Avoid walking or picnicking in long grass.
(e) Take seaside holidays rather than country, farm or walking holidays.

156 About 30% of individuals will get significant benefit from desensitization courses after three annual preseasonal sessions.

They are, however, expensive in both money and time, since they involve at least three visits to the doctor prior to the onset of the pollen season.

There is a significant risk of collapse, shock and sudden death and the doctor should have to hand adrenaline, hydrocortisone, O$_2$ and resuscitation equipment.

157    (a) First of all demonstrate the inhaler yourself using a special control aerosol.

       (b) Tell the patient to breathe out fully and then place the aerosol to the lips.

       (c) A slow inhalation is then taken, the canister being depressed once to release the aerosol during the initial phase of inspiration. There is no point in depressing the canister before inhalation unless a special spacer between aerosol and mouth is used.

       (d) The breath should be held for several seconds and then the air exhaled slowly. It is unnecessary to exhale fully as this may close off small airways.

In patients with particular difficulty then a rotohaler is useful as this is a simple breath activated device which delivers a measured amount of powdered drug.

158    In ordinary patients the dose of steroid produced by the body is constantly monitored and adjusted to suit the patient and in response to stimuli. Naturally most of the time a patient is not aware of increasing steroid demand unless the need is markedly increased and then it is too late for maximum benefit and suppression of the allergic response.

Steroid inhalers are also prophylactic and protect against a late allergenic insult. This can occur after 6 hours and up to 24 hours after an attack. It is, therefore, important to encourage the patient that these inhalers should be used continuously.

*Note:* if bronchodilator inhalers are also being used then the steroid inhalation should take place a few minutes after the bronchodilator aerosol.

159    (a) To assess the severity and reversibility of airflow obstruction using the peak flow meter. Effectiveness of bronchodilators can be checked with this instrument.

(b) To educate the patient and his parents or family about the nature of asthma, how to recognize the early signs of an acute attack, and the purpose, limitations and side effects of the treatment. When present, provoking factors should be discussed and possible solutions discussed.

(c) To discuss the long term prognosis and the possible effects in social and psychological terms, the ultimate aim being that the patient should manage his own illness.

(d) To rationalize drug therapy and to use as little as possible in as simple a regimen as can be arranged.

160 (a) That the patient and his family know and understand all aspects of the condition, treatment and general management.

(b) To improve as far as is possible the patient's ability to carry out ordinary tasks and functions.

(c) To prevent acute exacerbations but also treat early when they occur.

(d) To reduce the effort involved in respiration. This includes decreasing the production of secretions and improving elimination of mucus. Also reversible bronchospasm should be treated as far as possible.

(e) To reduce hypoxaemia.

161 (a) Unusual increase or decrease in the volume, consistency or colour of sputum.

(b) Sudden appearance of haemoptysis.

(c) Increase of shortness of breath or lethargy and general fatigue. In many cases the patient simply feels generally unwell and that he is going to be ill with headaches, dizzy spells, restlessness, lack of sexual drive or insomnia.

(d) Increased need for bronchodilators and more pillows on retiring.

(e) Onset or worsening of congestive cardiac failure manifesting as swollen ankles etc.

(f) Confusion, disorientation, sleepiness and often slurring of speech.

162 (a) The constitutional upset is very much greater than the physical signs or respiratory symptoms would suggest.

(b) The cases are occurring in epidemics when there are also occurring upper and lower febrile respiratory illness.

(c) When there is a history of contact with other sources of infections, e.g. pigeons, parrots or budgerigars in the case of *Chlamydia psittaci* or cows and sheep in the case of *Coxiella burneti*.

163 Very dangerous indeed. The average 'blue bloater' can suffer severe nocturnal hypoxaemia during sleep. This tends to occur during phases of REM sleep and is associated with transient hyperventilation and a rise in pulmonary arterial pressure leading to cor pulmonale. Hypnotics can increase the $P_{CO_2}$ and are therefore dangerous in these patients. Notable ones are the barbiturate group and the benzodiazepines.

164 First of all it must be remembered that medication should be given early. Do not await a sputum culture report with sensitivities. It is important to treat the patient immediately with a 'best bet' antibiotic such as co-trimoxazole or amoxycillin.

Because the illness is occurring in a lung which has been previously damaged then organisms of a normally less virulent nature can predominate.

If the patient responds in 3 days to the drug of first choice then there is no requirement to change antibiotics even if the sensitivities indicate that the organism is not sensitive to your chosen preparation. The major reason for the latter discrepancy is the difference between *in vitro* and *in vivo* results.

If there is no clinical response in 3 days then subsequent sensitivity tests are helpful and change to an appropriate antibiotic is indicated.

165 (a) Cigarette smoking—risks rise in proportion to the number of cigarettes smoked. Bronchial mucous glands become hypertrophied.

(b) Men suffer this illness more than women.

(c) An inherited tendency predisposes to chronic bronchitis.

(d) Areas of increased atmospheric pollution raise the incidence.

(e) Occupation—those in contact with smoke and noxious fumes have an increased incidence of chronic bronchitis.

(f) There is an increased incidence in social classes IV and V which is also linked with cigarette smoking. Winter months show the greatest morbidity and mortality.

166 (a) First of all the diagnosis must be confirmed and while doing this it is important to consider the alternative possibilities. These are:
   (i) tuberculosis
   (ii) bronchogenic carcinoma
   (iii) asthma—late onset type
   (iv) chronic left ventricular failure
   (v) other chronic chest disease, e.g. bronchiectasis and in the younger group, cystic fibrosis

(b) Once the diagnosis is confirmed then the degree of severity should be ascertained and monitored subsequently by chest X-ray—to exclude other pathology, e.g. carcinoma in heavy smokers. ECG should be done for evidence of RV strain. Lung function tests required are PEFR and FEV1. PEFR gives a good indication as to severity and progress. It will also indicate degree of reversible bronchospasm with the use of inhaled steroids, thereby indicating which patients will respond to corticosteroids either by mouth or inhalation.

(c) Any relevant risk factors should be defined and eliminated whenever possible, the main ones being:
   (i) cigarette smoking
   (ii) obesity
   (iii) occupation—discuss rehabilitation and retraining when relevant.

(d) Discuss the long term management with the patient and his family including home physiotherapy by the spouse during exacerbations.

(e) Drugs used include:
   (i) antibiotics—tetracycline and broad spectrum penicillins and co-trimoxazole during exacerbations. It is common for patients to keep a course at home for early use.

94

(ii) bronchodilators—only useful in reversible airways obstruction.
  (iii) corticosteroids—useful in asthmatic type if demonstrated to be of benefit.
  (iv) diuretics—helpful when cor pulmonale coexists.
  (v) oxygen—to be used sparingly and only when there is hypoxia.

(f) With patient deterioration then social services may need to provide home help, meals on wheels etc.

167 Yes, as follows.

(a) In patients who are hypoxic and who are experiencing dyspnoea due to this then $O_2$ relieves the severe breathlessness.
(b) Some mildly hypoxic patients find $O_2$ useful after exercise and it shortens the recovery phase.
(c) If used during exercise then exercise tolerance increases markedly.
(d) If used regularly in patients with cor pulmonale then mortality is reduced and there is a marked fall in pulmonary artery pressure and resistance.

The use of domiciliary oxygen is a decision which should not be made lightly as it is impossible to withdraw it once it has been used.

168 (a) A cough or recent onset without a febrile illness in all patients over 30 years of age. Later the cough has a 'brassy' characteristic.
(b) Haemoptysis—often an early feature due to erosion or fragility of blood vessels.
(c) Chest ache—this may be very vague at first, or can be severe due to a pathological fracture of rib or collapse of vertebral body. There may also be a general feeling of tightness or dyspnoea.
(d) Cyanosis and finger clubbing.
(e) Weight loss in someone with a normal appetite.
(f) Increasing shortness of breath with deteriorating exercise tolerance.
(g) Recurrence of chest infections particularly with localized chest signs or failure of one to resolve after antibiotics.

## J  Disorders of the urogenital system

169  Approximately 4–5% of disease presenting in general practice is related to the genitourinary tract. In any one year, given an average list size of 2400 each GP will see:

| | |
|---|---|
| Upper urinary tract infections | 25–30 cases |
| Lower urinary tract infections in adults | 30–40 cases |
| Acute genitourinary infections in children | 15–20 cases |

170  (a) Immediate microscopy provides an instant highly reliable test for urinary tract infection.
   (b) The test separates most true urinary infections from cases of urethral syndrome, thus providing a guide as to whether immediate antibiotic therapy will be of benefit.
   (c) The test will detect microscopic haematuria and detect other abnormalities such as hyaline or granular casts.

A drop of uncentrifuged urine is examined under high and low power for leucocytes (granular nuclei), red cells and bacteria. I use a counting chamber—not so much to actually count the cells but having to use a coverslip allows use of high power and when the grid is seen but no cells then one can at least be sure that the urine was clear and not that one failed to focus correctly.

If pus cells are present then the patient receives a 'best bet' antibiotic such as trimethoprim or amoxycillin. The urine is also cultured on a CLED slope in an incubator and positive samples sent to the laboratory.

If there are no pus cells then laboratory culture or negative slopes are awaited.

171  Urinary infections in young children can be very difficult to detect and may present as nausea and vomiting, failure to thrive or even a PUO.

   (a) Collect a clean specimen of urine. This ideally would be an MSU. In younger children disposable collecting bags should be used and the specimen brought to the surgery without delay.

(b) The urine should be checked for glucose and protein and examined for pus cells. When the latter are present they are highly indicative of urinary tract infection. Immediate culture on CLED slopes is advisable for maximum pick-up rates. Positive growth of single colony type should be sent for colony identification and sensitivities.

(c) If symptoms and signs (including the presence of pus cells) are indicative then treatment should be commenced while awaiting culture report. Appropriate regimens include amoxycillin, trimethoprim, co-trimoxazole or nitrofurantoin for 7 days.

(d) When infection is suspected then examine the child's abdomen and check the blood pressure with a paediatric cuff.

(e) Review the child after the antibiotic course and recheck the urine to assess cure.

In most cases referral for IVP and micturating systogram is made after one proven episode. This is because infection associated with vesicoureteric reflux can lead to renal scarring. Treatable congenital abnormalities are then corrected surgically and those not correctable surgically are at least brought to light and both parents and doctor understand the need for early antibiotic intervention in the future.

172 (a) Advise mother on hygiene and the need to cleanse the area around the prepuce. Emphasize, however, that she will be unable to do this until this infection has settled. It will help prevent further episodes.

(b) Regular retraction of the foreskin should be carried out. This should be done gently and the boy will eventually be able to do this himself.

(c) Check for an underlying cause such as glycosuria.

(d) Prescribe a 5-day course of amoxycillin or co-trimoxazole.

(e) Advise that, although circumcision is only occasionally warranted, it may be necessary if attacks continue.

173 Confirmation is by microscopy of the urine and subsequent culture. If there are pus cells in the

urine and the story is conclusive then commence therapy.

Infection is much less common in men and may be exacerbated by prostatic obstruction. Men over 50 should have an abdominal and rectal examination and ideally an excretion urogram to ascertain the degree of urinary obstruction.

The usual drug of first choice is trimethoprim for 5 days. This drug is concentrated in the prostate and helps sterilize the prostatic fluid as well as the urine.

174 (a) Poor standards of hygiene probably inter-related with lower social class lead to increasing numbers of pathogens in the area of the urethra.

   (b) Conversely too rigid attention to hygiene can provoke both urethral syndrome and acute cystitis. A deep bath forces bacteria loaded water up the urethra and the use of powerful bath foams can irritate the lower urinary tract.

   (c) Rough sexual activity can abrade the urethral meatus and allow ascending infection.

   (d) The presence of residual urine associated with bladder neck obstruction, calculi, divertula or vesicoureteric reflux can lead to acute cystitis.

   (e) Diabetes mellitus is a predisposing factor.

175 There are two main areas to cover, advice and treatment.

   (a) *Advice*
      (i) High fluid intake.
      (ii) Voiding of urine after bathing and after intercourse. The use of a shower is preferable to a bath. Also no bath foams.
      (iii) Improved local hygiene but not to use powerful disinfectants or perfumes or deodorizers.
      (iv) Remember to check for glucose as diabetics are more prone to urinary infections.

   (b) *Treatment*
      (i) Treat all acute proven infections with appropriate antibiotics.

(ii) Give her antibiotics to keep at home to take one tablet after bathing or having intercourse.

If not controlled then investigate with:

scan of kidneys and renal tract.
IVP.
micturating cystogram of residual urine if found on IVP.
cystoscopy.

176    First of all it must be remembered that proteinuria is quite common and does not always indicate renal disease.
    The Albustix method detects protein concentrations of 40 mg/litre and more. Normal urine contains 20 mg/litre. Because of this sensitivity, positives are common especially in alkaline urine. Conformation is necessary with sulphosalicylic acid (registers greater than 300 mg/litre) but may give positives in people on penicillin.
    A positive result should be repeated several times on early morning urine. If positives continue then an orthostatic test should be carried out:

(a)  urine voided on retiring,
(b)  urine collected on waking,
(c)  urine collected 2 hours after rising.

    If (b) is negative and (c) positive then an orthostatic cause is confirmed. If (b) and (c) are positive then further investigation is warranted. Remember protein excretion increases on standing for normal individuals as well as in disease.
    The next step is 24-hour collection. Normal amounts are less than $100 \text{ mg/m}^2$ body surface/24 hours. Greater than 200 is abnormal.

177    (a)  Orthostatic proteinuria which is exacerbated by strenuous exercise such as jogging.
    (b)  Any febrile illness can cause proteinuria.
    (c)  Following surgical operations particularly if these have been abdominal in nature or when blood transfusions have been given.
    (d)  Exposure to cold.

(e) Severe burns although these patients are transferred to hospital before proteinuria manifests itself.

178 (a) Feeling generally lethargic and listless with a chronic fever.
(b) Normocytic, normochromic anaemia due to haemorrhage, haemolysis or bone marrow involvement.
(c) Abnormal liver function tests by an unexplained remote effect of the tumour on the liver.
(d) Symptoms of malaise and weight loss due to 2° deposition in lung (cannon-balls) and bone.
(e) Erythrocytosis because of the increased production of erythropoietin.
(f) Hypercalcaemia which may be due to bony metastases or to parathormone production by the tumour itself.

179 (a) Haemoglobinuria due to strenuous exertion—March haemoglobinuria.
(b) The anthocyanins as found in beetroot and berries.
(c) Vegetable dyes used in colouring food.
(d) Cases of porphyria.
(e) Phenolphthalein present in alkaline urine.
(f) Heavy urate concentrations.
(g) Chemical and drugs such as phenindione and Pyridium.

180 The patient with renal failure commonly suffers from 'indigestion', ulcer-type pain and occasionally gastrointestinal bleeding. Some renal units actually give prophylactic cimetidine. The ideal treatment is simple antacids containing aluminium hydroxide or with added calcium.

Magnesium salts must be avoided as hypermagnesaemia can occur.

Cimetidine may accumulate and results in confusion. The normal maximum dose is 400 mg per day in any renal unit. In general practice this risk is too great to run and the product is best avoided.

181 (a) The rate of deterioration of renal function needs to be continuously assessed by checking serum urea and electrolytes and creatinine clearance rate. If there is an ac-

celerated course then there should be a search for correctable factors such as analgesic abuse.
(b) Blood pressure needs to be checked frequently and carefully controlled.
(c) Intercurrent infections and any stress such as surgery can cause either fluid overload or dehydration.
(d) Certain drugs are very susceptible to alteration in renal glomerular filtration rate and doses need to be modified accordingly. Common ones are digitalis, antibiotics and sedatives.
(e) If gastrointestinal symptoms develop then there must be strict control of dietary protein, perhaps down to 40 g per day.
(f) Calcium and phosphate levels must be monitored and controlled. It is essential that non-tourniquet samples be taken for this.

The early correction of phosphate levels delays the occurrence of renal osteodystrophy.

182 The use of immunosuppressant drugs naturally reduces the patient's ability to combat infection. Forty per cent of deaths in transplanted patients are due to infection. Widespread large warts can occur as can many of the common childhood infections such as varicella and indeed it can be fatal. Herpes zoster and herpes simplex infections are common and may cause systemic involvement with encephalitis. Obviously these patients should not be immunized with live vaccines.

183 The infection rate varies with the operator and is between 3 and 12%. There are two main areas involved:

(a) wound infection
(b) epididymitis.

They are roughly equal in prevalence.
Approximately 85% of the infections are endogenous due to bacteria present in the semen prior to vasectomy. The low incidence rate makes routine medication unwarranted and clearly automatic culture of semen prior to vasectomy is also uneconomical. It is, however, useful to remember this when explaining to a

post-vasectomy patient as the tendency is to blame poor surgical technique when this is not to blame.

184  A tight frenum and its tethering effect during penetration can cause pain during intercourse. This is secondary to stretching and tearing of the frenum during coitus. Circumcision is usually not required as the frenum can be lysed as an outpatient under local anaesthesia.

185  (a) Do not ask direct questions with yes or no answers. Ask open-ended questions such as: 'Have you noted any recent changes in your sex drive?' 'How have your relations been with your wife?'
     (b) Imply that you expect some difficulty to be occurring if they are feeling generally unwell, e.g. 'You must be feeling pretty low sexually as well.' 'I don't suppose sex has played a very significant part in your life recently.'
     (c) Avoid jargon or words which are too technical, e.g. 'Does premature ejaculation limit your coital activities?' Better to say 'Do you manage to come or climax at the same time as your wife?'
     (d) Try to avoid frightening words such as 'impotent' and 'frigid'.
     (e) Explore particular mentioned problems thoroughly.
     (f) Take time to listen without interruption.

186  Allergy to semen can occur and several cases have been recorded. The allergy is due to hypersensitivity to the seminal plasma and not to the sperms. One study showed prostatic extract to be the cause and IgE antibodies are responsible.

    Desensitization has been attempted but with mixed results.

187  There is no evidence that any particular food restriction is beneficial. Some advise against spiced food and curries in the belief that these irritate the prostate but there is no objective evidence.

    Heavy indulgence in alcohol can provoke acute retention of urine as can large quantities of tea and coffee.

Sympathomimetic drugs such as those found in proprietary cough linctuses can cause retention.

Useful advice to patients with mild hypertrophy is to avoid fluids 3–4 hours prior to going to bed. This often prevents nocturia.

In any year about three new patients will present with significant symptoms requiring treatment in a practice population of 2400.

188　The prevalence in the community is difficult to tell accurately and figures differ widely for patients over 65. The figures quoted vary between 10 and 45% for women and 10 and 25% for men. Up to 50% of patients admitted to acute geriatric units are incontinent of urine.

It is probably the single most important factor causing relatives to demand hospital admission for an elderly person.

## K  Disorders of the skin

189　Skin conditions are the fourth commonest diagnostic group encountered in general practice. With an average practice population of 2400 a general practitioner will see 300 skin conditions per year.

190　(a) The mode of onset of the condition and its progress since then.
(b) Has he noticed any factors in the environment which either alleviates or exacerbates the condition, e.g. is it worse or better at weekends?
(c) Previous problems with skin disease.
(d) Whether he has any systemic illness which may be significant.
(e) Any familial skin disorders or characteristics, e.g. atopy with bronchial asthma.
(f) Occupation.
(g) Details of any treatment used to date and how responsive the condition has been to its use.

191　Atopic eczema or infantile eczema can appear at any time in childhood but the most severe forms occur early. There is usually a family history of atopy, e.g. hay fever or asthma particularly in the parents. Persistent eczema is likely to be accompanied by the atopic syndrome. There are usually high IgE levels and multiple skin sensitivities on prick testing. Specific allergens are difficult to trace but in a few cases avoidance of cows' milk or egg improves the condition. Trials of this are worthwhile in selected cases.

192  This is a seborrhoeic eczema of the scalp which produces a thickened greasy flaking area.

The most efficient treatment is half strength salicylic acid and sulphur cream BPC nightly for about a week. Thereafter occasional applications may be necessary. The substitution of aqueous cream, as a cleanser, for soap is also beneficial.

193  The irritation is due to the breakdown of urinary urea to ammonia. This is exacerbated by residual detergent in the nappies and the greenhouse atmosphere of wearing plastic pants increasing the breakdown by skin flora. Once the skin is broken down the proteolytic enzymes and bacteria may be more irritant.

It is necessary to clean this skin throughly with soap and water and expose to the air as much as possible. Napkins should be washed with simple soap flakes only and changed frequently. Plastic pants are best only worn when the child is being taken out.

Topical barrier creams such as the following are helpful:

    zinc and caster oil ointment
    titanium preparations
    dimethicone and cetrimide ointment.

In resistant cases *Monilia* may be a secondary invader and nystatin cream can dramatically improve the condition and oral suspension as an adjunct is helpful.

194  This is how a cavernous haemangioma usually presents. It is not present at birth. It enlarges over the subsequent weeks and months reaching its maximum size by the age of one year. It can occur anywhere on the skin surface but if it occurs in the region of the orbit, anogenital regions or mouth it can cause problems with feeding, vision, excretion etc.

Over the succeeding few years the lesion regresses and is almost always cleared by school age. The disappearance commences by a whitening in the centre. There is no residual scarring.

Most mothers worry about bleeding but this is rarely a problem and surface pressure is all that is needed.

The main problem is convincing the parents that what appears to be a serious lesion will eventually regress without interference and that patience is all that is needed.

A useful adjunct is to take serial photographs of one child with a seemingly terrible haemangioma right from initial diagnosis to complete clearing. This set of photographs can be used thereafter for other concerned parents.

195 Most psoriasis sufferers are spared lesions on the hands and face but if these occur then there is a tendency for them to be photosensitive. Exposure to ultraviolet light in any form is therefore likely to cause a flare-up of the condition. In most cases, when thse areas are not affected the condition improves during summer.

196 (a) Have a bath before application, this prevents build-up.
(b) Apply 0.5% dithranol with 0.5% salicylic acid in equal parts of hard and soft paraffin to the area of psoriasis exactly. Aim for a local feeling of warmth. If burning occurs then stop for a few days. The psoriasis becomes thinner as a red-brown stain develops. The darker the better. The ointment is then covered with talc and old tights to prevent spread. If the lesions are small and widespread then micropore tape can be used.

The patient should wear old washable underclothes and use old bed-linen.
(c) When skin is smooth and does not flake when scratched, treatment can be tailed off.
(d) Staining can be removed with zinc and coal-tar soap BPC.

197 If only a mild burning is experienced this is acceptable. Here you must make some judgement about patient tolerance and maturity.

If there is real discomfort then use yellow soft paraffin for 2 weeks then resume dithranol 0.5% diluted with 4 parts yellow soft paraffin increasing the strength as tolerance develops.

198 There is no place for strong steroids in psoriasis. Initial improvement almost always occurs but rebound or early recurrence is common. Even worse, a plaque-like psoriasis may be converted to a widespead pustular or erythrodermic form.

199 The least potent corticosteroid ointment or cream should be used providing good control is achieved. Begin by using the mildest preparation and increase the potency to achieve a satisfactory response.

When potent steroids are used then more than 50 g per week produces measurable adrenal suppression.

If used sufficiently local effects occur namely striae, telangiectasia and atrophy. These effects are most marked where the skin is thinnest, i.e. face, flexures.

Areas with a thicker stratum corneum can tolerate higher doses as can the scalp.

When the lesion has settled then more bland preparations can be substituted such as:

   aqueous cream
   ung. aquosum
   Boots E45
   oilatum cream

Typical use is made of these in cases of atopic eczema in remission.

Remember! Never use steroids on acne rosacea, ulcers or superficial infections.

200 The most important lesions which can be treated in this way are cystic acne and keloid formation. In the past steroids have been used in this way for patches of alopecia areata but usually resolution occurs naturally. A rarer diagnosis is discoid LE but normally this is dealt with in the hospital situation.

201 Self-help includes a good wash with soap and water at least once a day. Shirts or blouses should be changed daily. The most satisfactory anti-sweating agent is aluminium chloride

hexahydrate but it is important to give specific guidance as to its use.

(a) It should always only be applied to dry skin as it is otherwise an irritant.
(b) Apply at night before retiring when sweating is less.
(c) Most patients find a small paintbrush the most useful applicator.
(d) Wash the skin the following morning.
(e) Apply every night unless the skin becomes sore and until the sweating ceases. When this point is reached then reduce the application to twice weekly and then once weekly.

202 Acne in an adolescent female is an embarrassing condition with occasionally very marked psychological sequelae. It is wrong to discuss the problem by saying it is a trivial self-limiting disease. With considerate sensitive management good results can be obtained. Mainstays of treatment are:

(a) general—scrupulous cleanliness of the skin using antiseptic soaps. Ultraviolet light at doses which are below that which would induce peeling are helpful.
(b) topical—sitting with a face over a bowl of steaming water softens the keratin plugs. Keratolytics may then be applied, e.g. 2% sulphur in calamine lotion building up to 4% as necessary. A newer product—tretinoin—is currently very popular, these should all be applied once daily.
   Local antibacterial agents which are also mild keratolytics are often successful, e.g. benyzoyl peroxide either on its own or combined with potassium hydroxyquinoline sulphate.
(c) Systemic antibiotics such as tetracycline 250 mg once daily can often induce remission but this must often be continued for several weeks.
(d) When cystic acne occurs then intralesional steroids should be considered for the larger cysts.

203 Most patients are aware that pigmented naevi can turn malignant and if they are numerous then the anxiety is proportionately increased.

Any pigmented lesion which grows rapidly in size, shows increasing melanin pigmentation, surface ulceration or spontaneous bleeding must be treated seriously. Urgent referral is indicated.

204 The rodent ulcer or basal cell carcinoma is the commonest form of skin neoplasm. They occur predominantly in patients over the age of 45 and whilst they can appear anywhere on the skin apart from the mucous membranes, and the palms of the hands and soles of the feet, the vast majority are on the face, head and neck. Approximately 50% of these are noticed by the doctor when the patient has appeared at the surgery for some other unassociated condition. On closer questioning the patient usually remarks that the 'spot' frequently scabs over and then breaks down. Only when the ulcer is very extensive does the patient complain of any symptoms. The early appearance is of a smooth translucent nodule which grows slowly and as it enlarges becomes depressed in the centre. A rolled edge develops with telangiectasia in the centre and on occasion there is pigmentation. In certain circumstances and when left untreated, large areas can be eroded away. The treatment of choice is X-ray therapy at the radiotherapy department which produces rapid healing. Excision can be carried out but this is rarely necessary. Recurrence is rare but follow-up is obviously advisable.

205 Obviously it is important to make a correct diagnosis since the treatments are very different. Problems both in diagnosis and treatment of skin lesions arise from the very thick stratum corneum in these areas in contrast to the flexures. Fungal infections of the feet usually involve the toe webs as well as the sole unlike either psoriasis or dermatitis.

206 Hypothyroidism—erythema abigne is a reticulated pigmentation of the skin of the lower legs because of persistent prolonged exposure to local heat. These patients frequently spend many hours in front of the fire holding a hot-water bottle next to the skin. This suggests that the patient feels the cold and this is a typical sign of hypothyroidism.

207   (a) General—look for exacerbating medical problems such as iron deficiency, anaemia, or diabetes mellitus.

    (b) Provide as much social support as possible by use of home helps, meals on wheels or even cottage hospital inpatient care to allow rest and elevation of the part.

    (c) Local treatment. If infection or pus is present then use an antibiotic which is active against the organism taken from a swab of the ulcer. Systemic medication is preferred and many clinics are also using metronidazole routinely in addition to main antibiotic. Local anti-infective agents such as povidone iodine can be painted on. When slough is present this can be dealt with using eusol and liquid paraffin. Benzoyl peroxide promotes granulation and is an antiseptic. Blue-line bandages are then used to wrap up the whole part. In hospitalized patients where facilities allow, pinch-grafting is performed to give skin cover. Dextranomer powder has recently been introduced and it is certainly very useful in intransigent cases but it is time consuming and expensive.

    (d) In some cases ligation of nearby varicose veins between exacerbations of ulceration prevents recurrences. Rarely amputation is carried out when ulceration is extensive and pain is a prominent feature.

## L   Disorders of bones and joints

208   Rheumatological conditions account for about 6% of any general practitioner's workload. In addition a further 6% is accounted for by trauma.

    In a practice population of 2400 in any one year a general practitioner will see the following:

| | |
|---|---|
| lumbago or back pain | 50–60 cases |
| prolapsed disc | 15–16 cases |
| sciatica | 5 cases |
| osteoarthrosis | 60–65 cases |
| rheumatoid arthritis | 12–15 cases |
| gout | 4–5 cases |

209   I.C.E. This stands for:

    (a) ice—or cold compress. With the six-fold increase in circulating blood volume more blood and tissue fluid are forced into the damaged tissue increasing pain, producing swelling and subsequent fibrosis. The cold compress should be applied for several hours. Ice out of the freezer should be protected from direct contact with the skin as burns may ensue.

(b) compression. The best system is cotton wool wrapped in crepe bandages or a double layer of tubigrip.

(c) elevation. This reduces tissue fluid collection by adding gravity to the natural flow forces. Tissue fluid is therefore reduced to a minimum.

These procedures are continued for 48 hours.

Some authorities also advocate the use of prostaglandin inhibiting drugs such as indomethacin thereby reducing pain production and vascular permeability.

Joint effusions if present should be aspirated as many times as necessary (under sterile conditions) and this also alleviates pain and reduces fibrosis.

210  (a) Absence of nerve root compression.
(b) More than one nerve root involved.
(c) Bilateral or symmetrical nerve involvement.
(d) Area of pain and tenderness is widespread and diffuse.
(e) The pain is continuous and does not settle when lying flat on a hard surface.

211  (a) He should have a firm bed, preferably with a board under the mattress to prevent the buttocks from sagging and increasing lumbar lordosis.
(b) When sitting, he should use an upright firm backed chair—preferably with arms. Low, easy chairs should be warned against.
(c) The patient should avoid lifting whenever possible. When lifting is unavoidable the legs should do most of the work and the back should remain straight. The patient should be shown how to lift with flexed knees and hips and a straight back with the elbows buttressed by the thighs.
(d) Weight control should be taught and an ideal weight calculated against age and height and sex.

212 Torn menisci are common. In any one year a general practitioner with an average list size of 2400 patients will see 15–20 cases. If the knee locks sometimes a general anaesthetic is necessary and arthroscopy is a useful diagnostic procedure.

Most minor tears will settle with I.C.E. and physiotherapy but approximately 10% will require meniscectomy because of recurrent locking, cyst formation or instability.

The long term effects should be explained to all patients considering meniscectomy as 85% will develop osteoarthrosis in 5–10 years.

213 Obviously since it involves looking inside the joint it will help establish a diagnosis when one is not clear. The most important indications are:

(a) Investigation of a monoarthritis of the knee.
(b) Diagnosis of unexplained synovitis.
(c) For obtaining a specimen for histology.
(d) The diagnosis or confirmation of a torn meniscus or other internal derangement of the knee.

214 (a) The toxicities of drugs used in this group of conditions are quite similar and are in some cases addictive. For instance a patient may be taking aspirin, indomethacin and prednisolone.
(b) Certain products can cause side effects such as peripheral neuritis (gold) or even myopathy (chloroquine and prednisone) which can appear to be a worsening of the original condition, the temptation then being to increase dosage with a consequent worsening of side effects.
(c) This group of patients has a high incidence of drug sensitivity because of the autoimmune basis of the original conditions.
(d) The chronicity of the underlying disease necessitates long term therapy.

215 Salicylic acid is rapidly absorbed from the stomach or duodenum. With a well recognized brand the rate of absorption is predictable and it begins within minutes and is completed in 3–4 hours. The physical characteristics of the

111

tablet, namely compression, coating etc. dictate the absorption rate.

In the body there is rapid hydrolysis in the serum and on reaching the liver it is conjugated by glycine and glucuronide. This conjugation has a maximum rate for any one person which on average is about 2 tablets per 4 hours, i.e. 12 tablets per day. When conjugation capacity is exceeded then toxicity results. In practical terms when no lab facilities are available, it is usual to give sufficient tablets to induce tinnitus and then slowly reduce until this symptom disappears. The limit of glycine conjugation has then been reached but not exceeded. The alternative is to check salicylate levels and maintain at 20–30 mg/dl.

216  (a) Establish a diagnosis before considering using the drug because once commenced it is difficult to diagnose the original condition and this drug is one which is difficult to withdraw.

(b) The initial dosage should be appropriate to the clinical situation. In acute episode of systemic lupus erythematosis it is usual to begin with a high dose but in say uncomplicated rheumatoid arthritis the dose is gradually built up until an acceptable dose limit is reached.

(c) With long term use blood glucose and serum electrolytes require monitoring.

(d) In ordinary individuals there is a normal steroidal release rhythm. It is illogical therefore to spread the doses throughout the day. Once daily dosage in the morning is appropriate.

(e) Because of long term side effects on the eye it is common to obtain baseline intraocular pressures and check for cataracts before commencing therapy. A local optician can perform this.

(f) Steroids suppress immune response and the patient should be counselled to report to you whenever he feels generally unwell. When you see him you should consider 'silent' infection as a possible cause for his symptoms.

(g) Patients should be given a steroid warning card to be carried by them at all times.

(h) Extra steroid dosage is required to combat

stress such as surgery or even a dental appointment. The patient should be made aware of this.

(i) When on large doses side effects such as myalgia, hypertension and oedema may appear to be due to a worsening of the disease. Be cautious about increasing the dosage and monitor the ESR as a reduction in therapy may be the correct course of action.

217 No. In the management of gout there are two distinct problems. First of all there is the excruciating pain of the monoarticular arthritis and there is the underlying problem of hyperuricaemia. These problems must be considered separately, however. It is believed that acute attacks are due to movement of the uric acid and treating the hyperuricaemia can aggravate or even precipitate an attack.

218 (a) The first step is to openly and honestly discuss the disease with the patient. The special areas to cover are how the disease will progress and how his life style may be affected. It is essential to maintain an air of optimism since improved management has now helped the long term prognosis.

(b) Promote daily exercise and physiotherapy to maintain mobility. Immobilization should be avoided if at all possible.

(c) Indomethacin and phenylbutazone have a specific anti-inflammatory effect. Suppositories for use at night can be particularly helpful.

(d) When there is marked hip involvement replacement arthroplasty may be necessary.

219 This simple investigation should be done on all patients with rheumatic symptoms. It will help pinpoint the occasional osteoarthritic patient who has in fact a different or additional diagnosis indicated by a high ESR.

In the elderly the three major causes of a high ESR are polymyalgia rheumatica, giant cell arteritis and multiple myeloma.

When a definitive diagnosis has been made then progress on treatment is monitored by the estimation of the ESR and a falling rate indicates improvement.

220   The most important diagnostic symptom is the voluntary statement of morning stiffness. In a typical case the patient complains of stiffness during the night while in bed but it is so marked on waking that they actually have difficulty getting out of bed unaided. In the more advanced but untreated case the spouse is involved each day. A hot shower helps and the morning activity relieves the problem. The stiffness may last one or two hours but can in the worst cases last all day. An accompanying symptom is what some authors call 'gelling', that is stiffening after resting for a while for example in a theatre or a restaurant.

221   (a) A high titre for rheumatoid factor.
     (b) The presence of rheumatoid nodules.
     (c) The systemic manifestations of rheumatoid disease namely malaise, muscle weakness, wasting and anaemia of the normochromic normocytic variety.
     (d) Presence of vasculitis.
     (e) Early appearance of bony erosions.
     (f) HLA-DR4 and or DR3 on blood testing. If these features are present then the patient's ability to cope must be assessed and you will need to come to some conclusion as to this ability in the context of social, psychological, physical surroundings.

222   At each visit during which gold is administered there should be an enquiry into aspects of reduced cell production, e.g. sore mouth, metallic taste or diarrhoea, also as to whether an allergy had developed, e.g. itch or rash. If an unusual symptom is described then the drug must be withheld.
    The following should be checked:

    (a) white cell and platelet count and haemoglobin.
    (b) urinalysis for proteinuria.
    (c) albuminuria—a low WBC count, sudden fall in haemoglobin, reduction in platelets and a rise in ESR are all indications to withhold the gold injection.

223   A chest X-ray. Bronchogenic carcinoma is commonly found presenting in such a way in this group.

224 (a) The most important single factor is to explain the nature of the illness to the patient. Many patients fear they have rheumatoid arthritis and it is important to allay this belief. It is important to explain that both rest and exercise must be taken in moderation and without excess.

(b) An ideal weight should be given and every encouragement offered to help the patient achieve this.

(c) Physiotherapy is helpful early in the disease and exercises help maintain muscle bulk. The meeting of fellow sufferers in the physiotherapy department can improve morale and help remove the 'why only me affected' syndrome.

(d) Heat treatment. Local heat can be very beneficial in reducing pain and stiffness.

(e) Aids and appliances are provided by the Department of Health and Social Services after advice from an occupational therapist. Home assessment may be necessary.

(f) Drug therapy—these are mainly analgesics and non-steroidal anti-inflammatory preparations. Intra-articular steroids in selected patients are helpful.

(g) Surgery—joint replacement is increasingly popular in producing pain-free mobile joints. Because of the increasing longevity of the substitute forms the trend is continuing.

225 (a) Reduced mobility—a mobility allowance will help a person to purchase and convert a car or allow the use of taxis to get about. A wide variety of wheelchairs are freely available. Concessional fares are available on public transport in many areas.

(b) Unemployment—if a person is classified as disabled it may allow him to be employed by a firm who by law must employ a percentage (4%) of disabled persons.

(c) Housing—if unsuitable this may be converted by social services or rehousing will be offered. A visit by an occupational therapist is necessary to assess functional impairment.

(d) Dependence—if sufficiently incapacitated then an allowance is paid to dependants or other persons supervising the disabled patient. The degree of incapacity must be very significant and is assessed by independent medical examination.

(e) Isolation—many professional and voluntary groups, some of a specialized nature, exist for support, e.g. Multiple Sclerosis Society, Age Concern etc. These can be coordinated through the Department of Health and Social Services.

## M  Disorders of the digestive system

226  Alimentary disease constitutes about 10% of a GP's workload. In an average practice list of 2400 patients the incidence of alimentary disease is roughly as follows:

| | |
|---|---|
| acute appendicitis | 3 or 4 cases per annum |
| renal colic | 3 cases per annum |
| biliary colic | 2 cases per annum |
| duodenal ulcer | 12 cases per annum |
| ulcer dyspepsia | 30 cases per annum |
| ulcerative colitis | 1 case per annum |
| strangulated hernia | 1 case every 2 years |

227  It is an important problem to identify pathological jaundice in the newborn. Physiological jaundice due to a rise of unconjugated bilirubin in the serum between the 2nd and 4th days of life can be aggravated by other factors. Any icterus occurring in the first 24 hours of life is pathological and usually indicates excessive haemolysis. If the infant is feeding poorly or shows any signs of abnormal behaviour then the bilirubin should be checked if jaundice is also present.

When the child is examined physiological jaundice does not extend to the lower abdomen. If icterus is present here and the baby was full term then this level of bilirubin is abnormal and the serum concentration should be estimated.

228  The routine treatment for this condition initially consists of simple measures, namely taking small meals, getting down to a normal

body weight, avoidance of food 4 hours before going to bed followed by antacids and elevation of the head of the bed by approximately 4 inches. If these measures have failed and there is considerable disability, repair of the hernia with the addition of other anti-reflux measures has a high success rate. In some cases poor results are due to inadequate screening of patients prior to the surgical procedure.

In others the digestive symptoms are not due to reflux and, therefore, not due to hiatus hernia, but are often coincidental in patients investigated because of dyspepsia.

229 (a) Immigrant children—particularly prevalent in inner city areas as outlined in the Black report.
(b) Alcoholics—this group use alcohol for calories and neglect food.
(c) Expectant mothers—may only clinically present when pregnant when the added stress is present in the form of fetal demand. A prolonged period of deprivation prior to pregnancy exacerbates the condition.
(d) The elderly—low income, poor motivation to cook for one or senile dementia are predisposing factors.
(e) Mentally ill—similar to (d).
(f) Patients with previous gastrointestinal surgery—malabsorption and intestinal hurry are the causes here.

230 In the treatment of peptic ulceration the use of antacids is one of the mainstays of treatment.
It is better to avoid calcium salt containing antacids for two reasons:

(a) calcium tends to cause constipation.
(b) calcium stimulates the release of gastrin and this may be an important consideration in ulcer perpetuation or formulation.

231 There has not been shown to be any benefit from advising patients to have the conventional gastric diet. They have no effect on gastric secretion and ulcer healing shows no acceleration. The major advice is to take small frequent meals of food of a type which the patient knows from experience will not upset

117

him. The effect of this is to help neutralize the acid. Fatty meals should be discouraged but the rationale behind this has not been worked out.

232  (a) It is imperative that the patient be seen promptly and a careful history and examination be made.

     (b) Admit to hospital all patients who have had an acute blood loss of more than a minimal quantity within the previous 48 hours. Prompt and adequate blood transfusion is the most important single measure in management. In the elderly the danger is even greater because of the risks of re-bleeding.

     (c) If the blood loss is trivial then in the first few days it is usual to enforce bed rest and give a light diet with a generous fluid intake to replace any loss. A haemoglobin check a few days later will validate the estimate of blood lost.

     (d) When the patient is known to have a peptic ulcer it is now usual to commence H2 blockers in full dosage.

        In cases of doubt or non-confirmation then commence antacids and arrange for a barium meal and endoscopy if available. In the very occasional case of heavy haematemesis or melaena then urgent gastrectomy is indicated when conservative measures fail.

233  (a) Any patient who is over 40 and complains of indigestion with anorexia and weight loss, particularly when pain is a feature.

     (b) A gastric ulcer which was considered benign but does not respond promptly to medical treatment.

     (c) Elevated ESR in the presence of anaemia and a positive faecal occult blood.

     (d) The recurrence of indigestion and weight loss after previous gastric surgery.

     (e) Vomiting due to pyloric obstruction or occasionally the presence of dysphagia due to lower oesophageal obstruction.

234  From a nutritional point of view this group of patients are at special risk from the following deficiency diseases:

     (a) iron deficiency anaemia

(b) B12 deficiency—occasionally folate also
(c) osteomalacia
(d) osteoporosis

In the present climate of use of H2 blockers gastric surgery is not common and the total numbers to be followed are not great. The general practitioner should therefore make use of a recall system either by use of a tagging display, disease index or computer record. Ideally patients should be seen annually, at least by the practice nurse. A system of picking up defaulters is necessary.

The following parameters should be observed and recorded and if necessary acted upon:

    weight
    haemoglobin and MCV
    alkaline phosphatase

Iron deficiency is in fact so common that many practitioners advocate routine iron replacement.

235   First of all it is imperative that the patient should understand what has been done to him and appreciate what the likely effects will be. This advice alone encourages patients to take frequent small meals. The symptoms are caused by the liquid meal being 'dumped' into the small bowel. The feeling of sweating, faintness and fullness are made worse by meals with hyperosmolar fluid.

Most patients obtain relief by taking their food dry and taking drinks separately and unsweetened.

There is no place for drugs. Occasionally a reversed jejunal loop has to be fashioned.

236   The two major identifiable causes of chronic pancreatitis are cholelithiasis and alcoholism. When alcohol is the cause then complete abstention, fat restriction and enzyme supplements can improve the condition markedly in 50% of patients. Supervision and frequent follow-up are the key factors in controlling alcohol abuse, but in those who default a miserable life is ahead.

Pain is a feature in about 80–90% of patients. The pain typically is epigastric and severe and occurs in bouts often penetrating through to the back. With continuing deterioration of the disease the pain lasts longer and is more severe. The pain may be aggravated by food or alcohol and when it wears off it leaves a dull ache. Heavy analgesia is often necessary and as a result narcotic addiction often ensues. This is aggravated by the personality types coexistent with alcohol abuse.

237 (a) Bilirubin, aspartate transaminase (AST), γ-glutamyl transpeptidase (γ-GT) and alkaline phosphatase. If these are normal then liver disease is extremely unlikely. A very high AST is indicative of acute hepatitis. A raised γ-GT indicates the possibility of alcoholism. An elevated alkaline phosphatase indicates obsruction in the biliary tree.
   (b) Urine bilirubin. If present then liver disease is confirmed and if the stools are pale then an obstructive lesion such as gallstones is most likely. If absent in a jaundiced person then this is suggestive of haemolysis.
   (c) Haemoglobin, red cell indices, and film. Target cells and spur cells indicate liver cell disease. A high MCV indicates alcohol abuse and the γ-GT should be checked.
      A low haemoglobin with low MCV indicates an iron deficiency anaemia and may be accounted for by blood loss from the bowel.
      A film may show evidence of haemolysis or a haemoglobinopathy.

238 There is no evidence that infection with hepatitis A virus progresses to chronic liver disease. There is a firm association between hepatitis B and active chronic hepatitis. There is now evidence that a non-A, non-B hepatitis causes chronic liver disease. This third form of hepatitis is the most common form of post-transfusion hepatitis in some areas.

239 The two criteria to be fulfilled are that the stones should be radiolucent and that the gallbladder should be functioning. The chemical is the bile acid chenodeoxycholic acid given daily and the patient is scanned at 6-monthly intervals. It works by reducing the cholesterol out-

put into the bile and causes the bile to be desaturated relative to the other bile lipids.

About 30% of patients have transient dose-related diarrhoea. The efficiency is reduced in obese patients and those on oral contraceptives and barbiturates.

If the stones are less than 15 mm diameter 80% of patients show dissolution in one year; if larger then the success rate falls to 25%.

240 (a) Anaemia—this is iron deficiency in type and usually slow and insidious in onset. When the stools are examined for occult blood then 10% are positive.

(b) Dyspepsia and change in bowel habit. In this group there is persistent pain and tenderness in the caecal area. Commonly there is accompanying nausea, dyspepsia and weight loss. The change in bowel habit may be a true persistent alteration from constipation to diarrhoea and vice versa or the symptoms may alternate.

(c) Abdominal mass. Approximately half the patients with this diagnosis have a palpable mass which may be the presenting symptom. Since the neoplasms of the ascending colon tend to be 'silent' for longer it is much more common to detect a mass in those carcinomas proximal to the hepatic flexure.

(d) Abdominal emergency. Some patients present with perforation and or peritonitis of the bowel and also as acute intestinal obstruction. The commonest area for this to occur is the sygmoid colon. Approximately 20% of patients present in this way.

241 (a) Eat a balanced diet containing cereal, wholemeal bread, fresh fruit and vegetables. Avoid too much white bread, pastries and sweets.

(b) If the diet cannot be changed then add one to two spoonfuls daily of Miller's bran on cereals or in soups, stews etc.

(c) Drink at least 4 pints of fluid daily.

(d) Take regular exercise.

(e) Always answer the call to stool promptly.

(f) Try to evacuate the bowels at a regular time but never sit and strain.

(g) Avoid long term use of stimulant laxatives such as senna.

(h) If all the above fail then use glycerine suppositories each morning to establish routine.

242  (a) Those with gross faecal impaction with or without an enlarged colon palpable per abdomen.
   (b) Any patient when rectal bleeding coincides with constipation.
   (c) Any patients with constipation and weight loss.
   (d) When symptoms interfere with social or family life and when they are taking time off work because of bowel disturbance.

243  Thirty per cent of patients of 60 years and over have evidence of this condition and it is already common in patients over 40 years. In fact the diagnosis of diverticulitis should be considered in any patient over 35 years with an acute abdomen.

   Treatment is with a high fibre diet, including Miller's bran. Since when loose it is difficult to carry, then tablets are useful substitutes. Other bulk forming agents are ispaghula and methyl cellulose.

   Initially two teaspoons of bran should be taken with each meal. Fluids must be taken at the same time. Bran can be added to cereals, porridge, soup, or sprinkled on ordinary meals.

   About half the patients feel bloated at first but this disappears gradually. After 2 weeks the amount of bran should be increased to produce one or two formed motions per day without straining. This latter point is very important as it shows that the viscosity of the original contents have been overcome and this reduces considerably the risk of haemorrhoids, irritable colon and diverticulosis.

244  In a typical case of Crohn's disease recurrent abdominal pain, diarrhoea and constitutional upset are the usual presenting triad. Sixty or seventy per cent do not have the constitutional disturbance and therefore when the abdominal pain and diarrhoea settle the diagnosis is not pursued in a proportion of cases. The 'dustbin' diagnosis of irritable bowel syndrome is then

attached to the patient and the correct diagnosis may not be made for many years.

245   It is now common for surgical opinions to be sought early so that the consultant can be involved at an early stage in the long term management. The main indications for surgery are as follows:

(a) failure to respond to medical treatment with a prolongation of symptoms and continuing loss of weight.

(b) management of complications such as a fistula or perianal disease.

(c) the removal of obstructing strictures.

In a recent survey it was found that in a large group of patients with Crohn's disease 70% had surgery for the condition during their lifetime.

246   Only the mild attacks can be treated in the home. A rough guide to this would be fewer than eight motions per day and when the patient is systemically well.

(a) Use oral prednisone in a dosage of 20–30 mg per day for adults. Continue for 4–6 weeks.

(b) Use a steroid enema (Predsol) daily until remission occurs and gradually tail off this drug depending on response. This may take 3 months. Be guided by clinical response.

(c) Commence sulphasalazine 2 grams per day. This should be continued indefinitely.

247   This drug should be commenced in the first attack and continued indefinitely. It is used to maintain remission and is effective over many years. In adults the optimum dose seems to be about 2 g per day.

   The active part of the drug is 5-aminosalicylic acid which is released in the colon. The other portion of the compound is sulphapyridine and it is this which causes the side effects of nausea, vomiting, sensitivity rashes and blood dyscrasias. The drug should therefore be continued indefinitely.

248   The practical procedure for changing the

appliance should be simple and quick. This helps the patient feel normal. It must be explained that the stoma may work erratically, particularly at first and that appliances may leak slightly from time to time. The skin surrounding the stoma should be washed with soap and water and using soft tissues the whole area dried. Avoid possible allergenic lotions or talc. Friction around the stoma may cause contact bleeding and this should be explained.

Odour and flatus can be very worrying. Putting deodorant in the bag can help and a filter allows flatus to escape.

Normal diet should be encouraged but it is important to explain that any abnormal foods such as curries can cause marked changes in habit, much greater than when the anatomy is normal.

Many stoma patients avoid onions or fish because of the smell they produce.

Encourgement to return to full activity is essential and normal work and hobbies should be restarted. Even food handling situations need not be avoided. Liaison with works doctors may be indicated here but only with the written sanction of the patient.

## N   Disorders of the eye

249   The approximate proportion is about 3% over a 12-month period.

With a practice population of 2400 a general practitioner is likely to see the following:

| | |
|---|---|
| acute conjunctivitis | 25–50 cases per year |
| styes (hordeolum) | 16–20 cases per year |
| corneal ulceration | 2–3 cases per year |
| acute iritis | 1 case per year |
| cataract | 7 cases per year |
| acute glaucoma | 1 every 2 years |
| retinal detachment | 1 every 3–5 years |

250   The wound in the cornea should be cleansed of imbedded foreign bodies. The first thing to do is to allow such an examination to take place. Pain is a prominent feature and it is necessary to anaesthetize the cornea with amethocaine. This should not be continued by the patient as it may delay normal healing. The area of the

abrasion can be delineated by the use of fluorescein stain. The impregnated papers are the easiest form to use and preferably should be moistened first before placing on the downturned lower lid. The stain is taken up by the abraded cornea and the damaged area inspected. After removal of any foreign material then chloramphenicol eye ointment may be applied and the eye closed and kept closed with micropore tape. Healing rapidly occurs with closed lids and the pain subsides. Complete rest for the eye for about 3 days is usually all that is necessary.

251 This is a light burn due to severe intensity of sufficient power to cause small areas of broken corneal epithelium. These result in superficial punctate keratitis. The pain is severe due to exposed nerve endings. The symptoms appear 6–12 hours after exposure.

The most satisfactory management is to close the eyelids with micropore tape and give potent analgesics such as dihydrocodeine or stronger. Since the lesion is sterile there is no need for antibiotics and complete rest for the eye is the main principle.

A similar ultraviolet burn occurs in snow-blindness.

252 These agents of which idoxuridine is the commonest are active against the DNA family of viruses, the major one being herpes simplex but also herpes zoster. The drops are intended for hourly instillation with the ointment being used at night. They act by inhibiting virus formation but also they affect the cells which are under attack from the virus itself.

Most experts would limit the instillation of these agents to 2 weeks as a greater use will damage the corneal epithelium.

253 This is a common condition whereby the patient feels as if there is something in the eye with a generalized grittiness or soreness.

The tear film covering the cornea consists of three layers. Directly on the cornea is a layer of water produced by the lachrymal gland. Covering this is a layer of mucus and overlying this a layer of oil both of which are secreted by the glands opening onto the lid margins and those in the conjuctiva.

The tear production fails when dry eye is present and this causes increased production of the mucous and oil layers which then stick to the conjunctiva and cornea.

Hypromellose eye drops ease the symptoms.

254 Spastic entropion. This occurs when there is spasm of the orbicularis musculature of the lid which turns the lashes inwards. It tends to affect the lower lid only and is not uncommon in the elderly. The inversion causes irritation of the eyeball and may even result in corneal ulceration. In milder cases the lower eyelid skin may be strapped down with sellotape but the more definitive operation is to remove a strip of lower eyelid skin.

255 Although eye drops are traditional and have been used for many years they are an ineffective way of supplying a high concentration of a required drug. It is unlikely that anything effective remains in the conjunctival sac for more than a minute after instillation. The exception to this are certain drugs such as atropine which are very rapidly absorbed through the cornea. The standard practice therefore of instilling drops three or four times a day serves no purpose. In severe cases, e.g. ophthalmic gonococcus, the drops should be instilled every minute and reducing gradually to every 15 minutes and sequentially thereafter for therapeutic levels to be maintained.

256 When the infection is mild then 'hot-spoon' bathing is usually sufficient. A piece of cloth or cotton wool is wrapped around a wooden spoon and immersed in water which is just hot enough to bear. The spoon is then placed in contact with the lid. This procedure should be carried out for about half an hour three or four times per day.

If there is marked cellulitis then add local chloramphenicol eye ointment four times daily and give systemic antibiotics. Since the usual organism is *Staphylococcus aureus* then phenoxymethylpenicillin or erythromycin are the antibiotics of choice.

257 It has been clearly demonstrated that long term systemic corticosteroid therapy can cause chronic open-angle glaucoma and indeed cataracts and in addition can provoke and exacerbate attacks of herpes simplex keratitis.

Local steroids are even more severe in their effects and have the added disadvantage of causing fungal overgrowth if the corneal epithelium is not intact.

258 There are two main causes for apparent squint. It must be extremely rare for there not to be some facial asymmetry in all members of the population. It does vary greatly between individuals. When this assymmetry is prominent the eyes can appear to be squinting.

Some children have exaggerated skin folds from the upper eyelids to the nose (epicanthus). This mimics a convergent strabismus. It is more prominent in individuals from the far east. As the child grows older then these folds recede.

259 When the visual activity is bad enough to interfere with normal life, e.g. reading a newspaper or seeing the television. The reason for not advising it earlier is that standard corrected vision after the cataract has been removed is very different and not as pleasing as substandard vision in an eye with normal anatomy.

Removing a lens and replacing it with a powerful spectacle causes a magnified image in a constricted visual field with no feathering at its peripheral edge. The result is a magnified world with images that enter and leave the field of vision without warning. For this reason an aphakic eye cannot combine with a normal eye to produce binocular vision.

260 Contact lenses are made from synthetic transparent materials and the eye accepts them only when there is adequate fluid exchange across the cornea and a plentiful supply of tears. Naturally there is fluctuation in fluid balance throughout the hormone cycle but it can be further unbalanced by pregnancy and the combined oral contraceptive pill.

Patients then complain of pain in the eyes on usual wear and this may become permanent should tear secretion diminish.

261　This point must be remembered. It may be due to extreme youth or poor intelligence or extreme misfortune. There are special checks for these two categories.

In the case of children the child sits on the mother's knee and observes a chart or cards of familiar stylized objects, e.g. car, house, cat, cow and he then points out which he 'sees' on a second card which he is holding.

With illiterate adults then the 'E' chart is used. Here the Letter E is presented pointing in different directions and in different sizes. Once again if they can demonstrate the direction of selected letters then it is assumed they are seeing this letter and the visual activity registered accordingly.

262　The principle here is to reproduce the characteristics of the pinhole camera. If you make a small hole with a large pin in a piece of card and the patient looks through this with both eyes in turn then visual activity can be tested. Because the field is limited it does not depend on lens qualities and therefore is independent of correcting lenses. This is a particularly useful method if you are suspicious that there is visual loss but the patient normally wears spectacles and has forgotten them on this occasion. It simply rules out spectacle error. If the macula has the potential to see a Snellen chart then the pinhole test will prove it.

263　This is a remarkably effective system of reading for the blind which was invented by a French youth aged 16 years living near Paris in 1825. His system was in fact an adaptation of a much more complicated system invented by Charles Barbier.

The braille characters consist of raised dots arranged in two columns of three. Permutations make up the alphabet.

$$1 \,..\, 4$$
$$2 \,..\, 5 \qquad \text{e.g. N} \,..$$
$$3 \,..\, 6 \qquad\qquad\qquad .$$

The system is very simple and blind children can read almost as fast as they can talk. Predictably blinded adults are slower to learn. The increasing use of auditory aids such as the 'talking book' are causing braille to be less well used, although in some countries such as the Netherlands all paper money has the denomination printed in Braille in the lower left-hand corner.

## O  Emergency situations in practice

264  Gastroenteritis is usually a short-lived disease and the vast majority of children are managed at home. Fluid and electrolyte balance is the most important factor in management. There are occasions when hospital admission is necessary:

(a) when moderate dehydration develops.
(b) when causes other than infection *within* the bowel are possible, e.g. meningitis, septicaemia, urinary tract infections, lower respiratory infections, otitis media.
(c) rarer medical causes such as haemolytic uraemic syndrome and cows' milk intolerance may present with diarrhoea and vomiting. The severity of the illness is usually a clue and the child looks ill and the symptoms have usually lasted several days with progressive worsening.
(d) surgical conditions can present in this way. Intussusception is characterized by colicky pain, a sausage-shaped mass in the abdomen and redcurrent jelly stools. Acute appendicitis is commoner in older children and may present with vomiting and diarrhoea.
(e) if intractible vomiting is preventing oral fluid replacement.
(f) if parental or other home conditions are inadequate, or when supervision is difficult in a clinically borderline case.

265  Shocked patients should ideally only be transported when they are stable and no longer in danger. This may mean erection of a drip and transfusing dextrose saline or plasma if more sophisticated plasma expanders are not available. Sometimes such replacement is not on hand or other life threatening conditions may intervene. Transfer of the patient to hospital is fraught with danger and the most important instruction is to insist on the patient being

horizontal for as much of the time as is feasible. Being carried head up can result in hypoxia to the brain resulting in unconsciousness and vomiting. Raising the legs in the early stages of shock can be helpful in improving the venous return. When carried head down the carotid sinus pressure increases which in turn reduces the peripheral vascular resistance and the end result is a further fall in blood pressure. The only safe solution, therefore, is to be horizontal in the 'recovery' position.

266 (a) Social deprivation with employment, poverty and poor housing.
(b) Social isolation from friends and relatives or where close support is lacking.
(c) Inadequate and aggressive parents often in social classes IV and V.
(d) Hyperactive or 'naughty' children.
(e) Unhappy marriage or history of divorce.
(f) The parents often come from aggressive families and they may have been abused themselves.
(g) Poor 'bonding' after delivery or separation early in the postnatal period. Battering is uncommon in breast fed infants.
(h) The injuries may be presented to the doctor late with inadequate explanation or sometimes overelaborate explanation.
(i) The child often appears developmentally retarded and indeed may be so. Failure to thrive is common.
(j) There is a suspicious manner in the child, a so-called 'frozen watchfulness'.
(k) Suspicious findings include multiple injuries over a wide time span, and injuries to relatively inaccessible parts of the body, e.g. genital area. Burns and scalds which are repeatedly occurring should alert you as the practitioner.

267 These occur mainly in elderly and are more likely to be present in those with borderline dementia. Their presence is related to poor oxygenation or limited cerebral reserve. The patient is restless, irritable and uncooperative. The fact that they are disorientated adds to their agitation and aggression. Understandably they feel they are persecuted and are often very frightened. There is often an underlying cause

and this must be searched for. The diagnostic possibilities are great and vary from acute respiratory infection to faecal impaction or urinary retention.

It is important to question the patient in a friendly sympathetic quiet manner. Try to appear calm and patient and do not lose your temper when they repeat simple questions. Take as full a history as possible, but often the story from relatives, neighbours and other persons involved are more important. Whenever possible refer to the patient's notes and look for potentiating factors including drug therapy.

Make as full an examination as possible although this may be difficult.

Try not to sedate the patient if possible as this may mask clinical signs and render diagnosis difficult. It may be imperative, however, if hospital admission is contemplated. If possible give oral drugs as this is not so frightening for the patient and more likely to be accepted.

Naturally if there is underlying disease this must be treated appropriately, e.g. with antibiotics in chest infection. If oral therapy is refused then admission may be warranted, especially if social circumstances are poor.

If home treatment is given then frequent follow-up is imperative. If sedation in the acute phase is indicated then use diazepam IV or IM (10–20 mg is adult dose) or chlorpromazine in age and size related doses.

268 Panic attacks are accompanied by highly intensive feelings of agitation. They are self-limiting and always acute. Occasionally there is an underlying condition such as temporal lobe epilepsy or phaeochromocytoma. It is often associated with hyperventilation producing faintness, tingling of the hands and feet and occasionally carpopedal spasm.

Reassurance and distraction may be all that is required. A firm kindness and interest in the patient produces the required atmosphere. If hyperventilation is present then rebreathing into a paper bag is necessary.

In the acute phase IV or IM diazepam (in adults) is beneficial and produces relaxation.

The use of beta-blockers such as propranolol in a dose of 40 mg thrice daily can prevent the somatic disturbance without producing drowsiness and these are useful as prophylactics when several episodes are occurring close together.

269 A suicidal gesture is always cause for concern and should never be treated lightly. It is usually a plea for help and this should be given not refused. If ignored serious accidents may occur if repeated.

(a) A careful psychiatric and social history is necessary. Such gestures are common in the young, in females, in those who are married and those in areas of social deprivation. It usually occurs after a 'lovers' tiff' and may be associated with taking alcohol.
(b) A personality study will usually reveal the patient to be attention seeking and manipulative.
(c) The patient should be interviewed with kindness and understanding and not with threats of police exposure or other displays of heavy-handedness. Having a combined consultation with the patient and spouse or boyfriend is helpful so that interpersonal stresses can be discussed.
(d) Social manipulation such as rehousing is sometimes necessary.
(e) There is rarely any place for medication, partly becuse there is none appropriate and also this would place the stamp of 'illness' on the patient.

270 Suicide is always a possible danger in depression and the doctor must make a careful assessment if the patient denies the possibility. It is usually held that the degree of self-reproach is an indicator, but the only true positive factor is that of a broken home in childhood. If suicidal thoughts are confessed to then admission to hospital is usually warranted because of the lag period for antidepressants. This is especially important where poor social circumstances prevail, e.g. being alone etc.

Parents occasionally fear they may harm their children. In most cases patients do not yield to obsessive impulses but this is an exception. Immediate admission to hospital is indicated.

271 All clothing except pants should be removed.

The room temperature should be lowered to 65–70°F. Aspirin 100 mg per day divided into 4-hourly doses or paracetamol 25 mg per day divided into 6-hourly doses should be given. If the rectal temperature rises above 103°F the patient should be cooled by tepid spraying until the temperature falls below 102°F rectally. Tepid water is less uncomfortable for the child and prevents vasoconstriction. One might suppose that fever control is sufficient to prevent seizures, but 30% of children with seizures associated with fever are not recognized as having a febrile illness beforehand.

All children with their first fit should probably be admitted to the paediatric unit. A lumbar puncture will exclude a CNS infection and a blood glucose estimation will exclude hypoglycaemia. The cause of the fever should be ascertained (usually viral) and treated. It is important that parents be taught the first aid aspects of managing a child with a seizure.

If decided upon then seizure prophylaxis should be commenced and continued for 3 years or until the child is 5 years old (whichever is shorter).

General management guidance consists of advising copious fluids until the child is hungry and slowly reintroducing solids thereafter. Rest is recommended until the child is afebrile.

272 Most convulsions are self-limiting, but every attempt should be made to stop seizures which are not self-limited within 10 minutes.
 (a) Place in the recovery position.
 (b) Ensure a good airway.
 (c) Intravenous benzodiazepines e.g. clonazepam 1 or 2 mg or diazepam 0.3 mg kg.
 (d) Intravenous infusion into a convulsing chubby infant is not always possible. Then it is best to give 2–5 mg of rectal diazepam via a needle-less syringe or 2–5 ml of paraldehyde by deep intramuscular injecton. All things considered the rectal diazepam is the best and easiest choice for although it is possible to use plastic syringes with paraldehyde if used immediately it is still a painful injection.
 (e) If the child does not settle rapidly or the social circumstances are poor then admission to hospital for observation is indicated.

(f) Make sure that close supervision for the rest of the day is possible as the most common time for a repeated convulsion is closely following an initial attack.

(g) Make arrangements to revisit the child that day and counsel the parents regarding first aid measures during seizures.

(h) Consider long term prophylaxis.

273 (a) One would admit a distressed child who is restless and pale or cyanotic with clinical signs in the chest, either wheezes or crackles.

(b) If there is both inspiratory and expiratory stridor then suspect epiglottitis especially if the child is febrile, obviously ill and drooling. In these cases do not inspect the throat as depressing the tongue can completely obstruct the airway.

(c) Poor social conditions or where the parents are inadequate would indicate admission to hospital. Where there is extreme anxiety in the parents it is unlikely they will be calm enough to provide the restful atmosphere necessary for nursing these children with water vapour inhalations.

274 (a) The story may be a reasonable one but the ECG does not change over a few days. It is important to treat the patient clinically rather than from an ECG reading.

(b) The pain may occur in an unusual site, e.g. upper abdomen or jaw.

(c) The pulse, B.P. and other initial signs may remain absolutely normal after the attack.

(d) There may be no pain at all in the chest but the patient may merely faint or develop acute left ventricular failure. This is due to the onset of an arrhythmia. The diagnosis is confirmed by ECG and enzyme studies.

275 ECG studies reveal that almost all cases of acute myocardial infarction show arrhythmias in the early stages. Extrasystoles are the most common and often lead to more sinister complications so obviously early treatment is indicated. Supraventricular extrasystoles are premature beats without a full compensatory pause and they are relatively benign and require no treatment. Ventricular extrasystoles,

however, have a full compensatory pause and are significant as they predispose to ventricular tachycardia and then on to fibrillation. 100 mg of lignocaine intramuscularly is the drug of choice for ventricular extrasystoles but if the patient is hypotensive this injection should be given intravenously and slowly.

276 (a) The patient is in stable sinus rhythm with no conduction defects, arrhythmias, frequent extrasystoles and is not shocked.
(b) Patient's desire and relatives' agreement.
(c) Adequate medical cover available.
(d) Good support from other primary care team members and family.
(e) Onset of symptoms occurred at least 4 hours prior to doctor seeing the patient.
(f) Chest pain controlled in 24 hours and no intractable heart failure.
(g) No relevant past medical history which will complicate the picture.

277 (a) Any patient who is severely ill with typical signs of tachypnoea, central cyanosis, dehydration, hypotension, jaundice, restlessness or altered consciousness.
(b) In cases where there are unsuitable social or domestic circumstances, e.g. poor housing, no relatives etc.
(c) When pneumonia occurs secondary to some primary lung disorder such as influenza, airways obstruction, cor pulmonale. A rarer occurrence is when the patient is on some preparation which reduces the body's defences, e.g. immunosuppressants for neoplasm.

It is common, however, for pneumonia to be a terminal event in most illnesses and this will naturally modify any proposed transfer. Do not deny the right for the patient to die at home looked after by his family if this is appropriate.

278 (a) There is use of accessory muscles of respiration with marked difficulty in speaking.
(b) Sudden decrease in exercise tolerance.
(c) The PEFR drops markedly to less than 120 l/min.
(d) There may be so little air entry that wheezing cannot be heard and the chest remains

135

overinflated. This is due to a combination of bronchospasm and mucosal oedema. The result is the 'silent chest'.

279 (a) The presence of haemoptysis or blood stained sputum suggests acute lobar pneumonia, pulmonary infarction, tuberculosis or neoplasm.

(b) The onset of pleuritic pain—sharp chest pain in relation to breathing movements or change of posture. Often found in pulmonary infarction, lobar pneumonia, plurisy, bronchogenic carcinoma and myocardial infarction.

(c) Fever greater than 5 days' duration with or without antibiotic intervention. The likely causes now are virus pneumonia, resistant bacterial pneumonia, neoplasm underlying or tuberculosis.

(d) Systemic effects, e.g. rapid respiratory rate (greater than $20/\text{min}$), restlessness, pallor and in babies intercostal recession.

280 (a) Usually the patient responds in a few days after ingestion of a drug to which they are sensitive. If the drug has been given before then the reaction may be immediate. Occasionally a reaction can occur several days after a course of treatment has finished or even during prolonged use.

(b) Check if the patient has had a similar episode previously. Recurrent eczema or psoriasis can complicate the diagnosis.

(c) Patch testing is not helpful and can be positively dangerous. Intracutaneous prick tests are helpful in investigating penicillin allergy.

(d) All drugs should be withdrawn or substituted. This is best done in a sequential way to reduce problems of medication supervision. When the rash settles, if reintroduction is essential, then the patient can be rechallenged using a very much lower dosage. This should be done under supervision and if all resuscitation facilities are to hand, but even then only if the reaction was *not* life threatening.

281 The majority of acute back problems have no underlying cause and usually follow a lifting-

twisting injury. Ninety per cent recover with simple measures in 2 or 3 weeks. They tend to be recurrent and most commonly occur in the 30–60 year age group. The first step is to advise strict bed rest on a firm base for 2 or 3 days with aspirin or paracetamol for analgesia. The firm base may be the mattress of the bed laid directly on the floor or boards inserted under the mattress.

After 48–72 hours the situation must be reassessed. Check for bladder function, ankle jerks or increasing pain particularly if only one leg is involved. If the signs are indicative or if pain is not under control then urgent referral is indicated because of nerve root compression.

Possible future treatment involves epidural anaesthesia, manipulation, pelvic traction or surgery after myelography.

It is important at the outset not to miss the serious signs of nerve compression namely loss of sphincter control and unilateral absent reflexes.

282   The important principle is that they should be removed completely and painlessly and any resultant ulcer or abrasion should heal completely.

If the foreign body is in the lower fornix this can be removed by a cotton bud soaked in saline.

In the upper fornix the foreign body is removed after eversion of the lid.

When the foreign body is embedded local anaesthesia with amethocaine is indicated. The most satisfactory instrument for removal is a large gauge sterile syringe needle. This should be performed in a good light with adequate magnification.

Any remaining ulcer will be demonstrated with fluorescein. Some authors advise a mydriatic be used for a few days, together with a topical antibiotic such as chloramphenicol. The quickest way to heal such an ulcer is to give complete eye rest by closing the lids with micropore tape.

If the foreign body was metallic then any remaining rust stain should be carefully removed usually at a later date.

283   The usual cause is direct trauma. The orbit

provides good protection but some missiles are too small to be deflected, e.g. golf balls, squash balls, shuttlecocks. In these cases the eye receives the direct blow.

First of all check that the patient still has vision in the affected eye. This may mean prising open the oedematous lids. Visual acuity may be examined then in the usual manner, i.e. Snellen charts.

Check the following: integrity of cornea and anterior chamber; look for hyphaema; does the pupil react?

Next examine the fundus as damage to the retina if it occurs can be permanent.

The ocular movements should then be examined. If the eyeball has been driven back the bony orbit gives way in the floor. The result is a restriction in elevation.

Finally look for any 'stepping' of the bony orbit which might indicate fracture.

284 This is due to the restriction of outflow of aqueous from the eye and it is precipitated by pupil dilation. The condition is more common in hypermetropes because of the shallow anterior chamber. The typical symptoms are:

(a) severe deep throbbing pain which may radiate within the distribution of the trigeminal nerve.

(b) greatly reduced vision at the time of the attack. There may be premonitory symptoms such as haloes as the pressure begins to rise.

(c) nausea and vomiting may be so severe that you will concentrate on these first before recognizing the true diagnosis.

(d) watering of the eye.

285 The general principle is that the coroner should be informed whenever there is any doubt as to the cause of death.

The statutory categories are:

(a) death occurring more than 14 days after last attending the patient.

(b) death when the doctor has not been attending.

(c) death to which an accident has some contributory part.

(d) cases of violent death.

(e) circumstances of doubtful stillbirth.

286   (a) The assessment of the patient's problems should be accurate and comprehensive.

      (b) The patient should feel that the doctor has evaluated his problems accurately.

      (c) An appropriate management plan should be constructed which is satisfactory to both patient and doctor. This should also be realistic in terms of cost, time, risk, possible conclusion.

      (d) The time used should be economical and effectively managed.

      (e) The outcome should be satisfactory for both patient and doctor and the relationship enhanced.

287   The interpretation of physical contact varies with different cultures but when a doctor touches a patient or vice versa then protection or empathy is being sought or given.

    During the examination then touch by the doctor is acceptable and this conveys psychological benefit. Subjective benefit measured by patients after a consultation has been shown to be improved if physical contact has taken place.

288   (a) The more medical knowledge a patient has then the more he will retain.

      (b) The more a patient is told then the greater the proportion he will forget. Ley and Spellman* found that only if true facts were given was recall good.

      (c) Patients who are mildly anxious will retain more than either those who have no anxiety and those who are extremely anxious.

      (d) If advice is given appropriate to intelligence and social class and amplified with diagrams and guidance leaflets then retention is improved.

      (e) What patients are told first and last are retained best of all.

    The motto should be tell patients no more than four facts. The beginning of the advice should be a summary followed by more detailed information including diagrams and leaflets and ending with a summary of the four main points.

* Ley, P. and Spelman, M. S. *Communicating with the Patient* (London, Staple Press).

289 (a) Self-employed men or people in responsible situations. Here job priority over
health is common. This is continued in the
tendency to return to work as soon as
possible and sometimes too soon. Here you
should be aware once again of the minimiz-
ing of symptoms.
(b) Patients who are used to pain and discomfort. Commonly the doctor is called only
after the pain has been present for some
time. This is common in the elderly when a
broken neck of femur may have occurred
several days earlier.
(c) When there is fear of serious illness a
patient will sometimes stay away until the
last possible moment. An example here
would be a lady with a large breast carcinoma which she has noticed for several
months.
(d) Some patients with medical knowledge
may falsely diagnose their symptoms as
being less serious than they really are or
present late because of fear of appearing
neurotic. It is common for midwives to
present to the labour ward in advanced
stages of delivery because they fear it may
have been a false onset of labour and thus
they would lose face before their peers.

290 Guilt usually occurs when we have failed per-
sonally. Typical examples are as follows.

(a) A relative of an elderly person demands
that something must be done immediately
to get the patient into geriatric care. Often
this is because the younger relative feels
guilty that he could, but won't do more,
albeit with some extra effort on his part.
(b) A common time for a doctor to be called is
when a husband returns from work to find
a child has been unwell all day. In this case
the mother will ask for a late visit and she
feels she has neglected the child by not
calling the doctor earlier.
(c) Many patients feel guilty about calling the
doctor out at night. In this situation the
relatives usually ask 'Did I do right in
calling you out doctor?' Another situation
is when a patient feels that he has gone
against accepted custom, e.g. a child is able

to fall into a unprotected fire or take an overdose of easily reached tablets.

In order to expiate guilt then patients may distort the facts to make a visit to the doctor or a night call more justifiable.

For example: a mother of a child with recurrent urinary infections rings for a late-night call from her general practitioner. On arrival he is told that he has said she should call him out *immediately* there was a recurrence of the urinary infection.

291　When a patient seeks medical advice he is admitting he needs help and he has accepted the role of a sick person. He does by this act lose independence and becomes dependent upon the doctor and his own family. The full definition is the reversion to behaviour patterns which were normal at an earlier stage of development. Some degree of regression is helpful to recovery, i.e. listening to and acting on advice from others. As the patient recovers then increasing independence is allowed by the doctor.

If regression does not occur then they may fail to follow treatment or there may be a denial of illness.

If excessive, then the patient is very demanding of medical help and recovery is often slowed. Usually the underlying cause is fear of the diagnosis or the thought that they are not being told everything.

292　(a) At the end of the consultation the doctor stands but the patient remains seated.
(b) The patient suggests a further investigation or a hospital outpatient appointment.
(c) The patient brings a relative into the consultation and this 3rd party may ask searching questions obviously on the patient's behalf.
(d) Even after what appears to be an adequate explanation the patient requests more information about his problem.
(e) Before leaving, sometimes on leaving (door-handle complaint) the patient makes a remark that they are obviously unhappy about the advice they received or by the nature of the question the advice is not acceptable.

293　The most important risk is that an organic disease

may be missed because of concentration on psychological factors. Anxiety and organic illness frequently coincide and it is important to sort out which is the most important factor in each case.

Many young practitioners concentrate wholly on one aspect or another. The danger of emphasizing the organic aspects when this is not the underlying cause is that a doctor's obvious preoccupation with the organic symptoms underlines the patient's anxieties about the seriousness of the situation. At the end of the consultation, especially if extra tests have been arranged and no reassurance given, then the suspicions of a patient are virtually confirmed by the doctor's concentrations on the organic nature of the case.

Perfection, if achievable, is a balance of physical, pschological and social aspects.

294 These are all examples of occasions when there is a change of role on the part of the individual. Some people accept the change readily and because there is a measure of choice in some of them then acceptance is implicit. Not always is the change of role fully understood and then this situation has potential problems. When some of these changes are forced then more problems are likely to arise. Previous personality and the abruptness of the change are two valuable predictors as to outcome.

295 Aggressive behaviour displayed either by doctor or patient can only be harmful in any consultation. The patient furiously justifies or attempts to justify his reasons for coming and this distorts the true story. It leads to a misinterpretation of the clinical facts and the social and psychological factors which have brought him to the consultation.

The result will then be either a false diagnosis or an unsatisfactory management plan. There may be unnecessary investigations and deferral or lack of the same when these would be appropriate.

It is important to recognize the aggression objectively and to analyse the cause. When this is done the situation can be defused and satisfactory objectives for both patient and doctor can be achieved.

296  This is the degree to which patients follow advice given by their doctor and other members of the primary care team. There are many factors which influence this, some of which are as follows:

(a) a patient's satisfaction with the doctor and also with that particular consultation.
(b) if the condition for which advice is being sought is causing a significant degree of disability then the patient is more likely to follow reasonable advice.
(c) a simple drug regimen or small change in behaviour is more likely to be followed than more radical changes which would affect the patient's whole life, e.g. giving up smoking, losing weight, complicated and unpleasant drug regimens.
(d) the amount of interest taken by the doctor in the patient's health affects whether he will follow advice given and, therefore, frequent follow-up appointments can be significantly helpful in improving patient compliance.

297  (a) The major cause must be husband/wife incompatibility due to an initial poor selection with progressive worsening of the relationship.
(b) If the husband or wife works a great deal away from home then communication breaks down and alternative mates are sought.
(c) Male domination is to a large extent diminishing and independent ladies are now not prepared to accept without debate what their husbands consider to be their lot.
(d) The press and media give young couples expectations for marriage which are excessively romantic and not realized.
(e) Many couples now move out of their home area. When problems arise there are no moderators nearby to help discuss the problems with maturity.
(f) Fewer children are now being born to young couples. This leaves the wife with more free time. In addition divorce is less harrowing.

(g) Divorce as an entity is now more widely accepted and couples who would in the past have stayed together because of social pressures are now separating more quickly.

298 The four main areas other than the obvious symptoms are:

(a) marriage—marital conflict or boyfriend/girlfriend breakdown can have far-reaching effects. These are not often discussed ab initio but should be explored.
(b) family—worries about children's futures figure largely in the lives of most adults. There may be anxieties over school acceptance, job opportunities, conflict with the other parent, adjustment to adolescence etc.
(c) friends and outside interests—sometimes worries about physical disease affect friendships and certain illnesses have a stigma attached which can alter attitudes to mixing with peers.
(d) occupation—problems of an interpersonal nature at work have reverberations within the other areas. Arguments with workmates can affect behaviour.

299 When subjected to stress all humans respond physically and mentally. The degree of response depends on the two variables, (a) the person's particular resistance to stress, (b) the severity of the stress.

The three levels of response are:

(a) anxiety. Mild stress produces apprehension but when increased there are symptoms of 'free anxiety' which includes palpitations, anger, depression, loss of speech control. Physical effects include raised heart rate and pulse rate, respiratory rate and metabolic rate. There are actually changes in urine, blood and saliva.
As the stress increases panic ensues and this usually ends in inactivity.
(b) conversion. Certain aspects of anxiety are converted into bodily symptoms which cannot be objectively validated by the doctor. One effect is that the patient may use

144

these anxiety related symptoms to justify his attendance at the surgery.

(c) physical disease. This is true psychosomatic disease when stress actually causes disease in the tissues. The target organs vary but examples are ulcerative colitis, duodenal ulcer, angina pectoris, dermatitis artefacta.

300   There are three stages. The initial stage can last for hours or even a number of days. The beginning is immediately after death and at first the patient is numbed and with this feeling there are outbursts of anger and extreme distress. There is often, at this stage, a period of denial of the event having occurred.

An intermediate stage is one of painful pining and the events leading up to the death are recalled. This stage is accompanied by a strong impression of the dead person's presence and this can be alarming to the patient. Over the succeeding 2 weeks these feelings diminish in intensity. There is often a desire to blame someone for the death of their loved one and, in some cases, this guilt may be self-directed.

The final stage can last for up to 18 months and consists mainly of depression and apathy and the loss of a specific purpose in life. Typically, by the end of the second year after death, it is normal for life to become reorganized and the whole experience more acceptable.

301   (a) When the bereaved has developed symptoms similar to the illness which caused the death of his partner.

(b) Strong feelings of self-blame attached to the death, e.g. sending into hospital.

(c) Depression so severe that suicide has been attempted.

(d) Cases of sudden death are related to poor resolution of the grief state.

(e) Bitterness, paranoia or resentment at being left behind.

(f) No obvious emotion at all about the death or in fact wandering aimlessly about and not partaking of social opportunities offered to them.

(g) Constant pining which interferes with everyday living.

302   In most cases this family has lived in the area for

several years and usually extends to many relatives in the town or nearby area. These relatives are a source of advice and disharmony, e.g. mother-in-law living across the road. Usually the roles of all members are fairly well laid down.

The father is the wage earner and most of this income is used to feed and clothe the family. He tends to go out drinking at weekends perhaps occasionally with his wife. Mother is often in charge of the detailed financial affairs and she does not expect her husband to help with the housework.

Children learn to be dependent on the others for support and in large families the older female children bring up the younger ones to a large extent.

Behaviour problems are common but often never reach the consultation because they are dealt with within the family framework.

Materialistic attitudes are often only extended so far as owning a television or a car.

Violence in such a family unit is common and often accepted by all members.

303  (a) When a serious illness is diagnosed in a hospital patient the GP should be contacted as soon as possible by a senior member of the team.

(b) A detailed discussion should take place between consultant and GP to review all aspects of the disease. The consultant would gain relevant social and family details and the GP will be informed of the immediate management.

(c) A home visit by the GP to the family is helpful to discuss the significance of the illness and to answer their queries.

(d) When the patient returns home then a detailed discussion between GP and patient should be offered although this may be rejected.

(e) The GP should have an outline of the proposed management plan with details of future investigations and drugs used. Whenever new drugs or regimens are tried then side effects and points to watch for should be included, plus a realistic prognosis.

(f) The line of communication between GP

and consultant should be maintained and any new developments in the patient's condition should be discussed.

This feeling of working together significantly boosts the morale of the patient and his family.

304  (a) *Alcohol*

(b) *Hypnotics, sedatives and anxiolytics*, e.g. amylobarbitone and chlordiazepoxide

(c) *Antidepressants*, e.g. amitryptiline

(d) *Neuroleptics*, e.g. chlorpromazine and haloperidol

(e) *Antihistamines and anticholinergics*

(f) *Analgesics*, e.g. codeine and deeteropropoxyphene

(g) *Anaesthetics*

(h) *Amphetamines and cannabis*

(i) *Phenobarbitone*

(j) *Hypoglycaemics*

# HUMAN DEVELOPMENT

305  Almost all general practices have a stable population of approximately 2400 patients per doctor. There is greater patient mobility in city centres and dormer suburbs and less in rural areas. This allows long term research and health prevention programmes to be carried out.

Patients visit their doctor for various reasons during the year and these incidental contacts provide opportunities for health education and screening whatever the presenting complaint may be. Ninety-five to ninety-seven per cent of patients will see their doctor in a 5 year period.

The overall consultation rate throughout the country is 3–4 contacts per annum. It is greater for mothers with children (5 or more contacts per annum) and much less for adult males of the 20–40 age group.

306  (a) To help the child establish both active immunity against specific infectious diseases namely measles, pertussis, poliomyelitis, tetanus and diphtheria.

147

(b) To screen for specific diseases and conditions which if detected at an early stage or prevented altogether significantly affect the child's development and future health. Examples are phenylketonuria and congenital dislocated hips.

(c) To help a child achieve optimum development both physical and mentally.

(d) To help the family adjust to the child's presence and integrate the infant into his relationship with the other family members.

307 (a) Pregnancy. In this case the immune response by the fetus is inadequately developed and spontaneous abortion or miscarriage may occur.

(b) During an established febrile illness. Here the immune response will be 'distracted' and immune reaction possibly muted.

(c) When the patient is on systemic steroids.

(d) During and after courses of immunosuppressant therapy.

(e) After courses of radiotherapy.

(f) Where the body's immune response is otherwise abnormal either congenitally due to hypogammaglobulinaemia or secondary due to carcinogenesis.

308 (a) If the child has an acute febrile illness at the time of proposed immunization.

(b) Any abnormality of the central nervous system.

(c) History of previous convulsion either febrile or not and particularly if there were signs of cerebral irritation in the neonatal period.

(d) If there has been a general or local reaction to previous immunization attempts.

309 (a) When given a small toy then some attempt at examination is made by the infant and when dropped, as usually occurs, then it is looked for.

(b) If given something edible such as a rusk then he will attempt to feed himself. He will also be able to drink by himself from a cup albeit imperfectly.

(c) When a sound is made he will turn towards the source and localize accurately.

(d) The child himself will have begun to mobilize and be able to make at least three distinct sounds.

(e) When placed on his back he is able to roll unaided into the prone position.

(f) If sat in an upright position he is able to hold this for several seconds unsupported.

(g) When held by mother in a standing position he will bounce up and down.

310 This is a chart with two axes namely length or weight against age, such as the ones designed by Tanner and Whitehouse. Body measurements for a given age vary from person to person for a number of reasons, including inherited constitution, dietary factors, specific illnesses and emotional deprivation. The distribution of such measurements of children at each age is expressed in percentiles. Any particular percentile refers to the position which a measurement would hold in a typical series of 100 children.

The 10th percentile is the value for the 10th child in a series of one hundred if arranged in rank order with the least being number one, i.e. 90 children in the series would be larger in the parameter measured. The 50th percentile is the median position.

From the point of view of normality the 97th and 3rd percentiles mark the boundaries of normality. It is of particular importance to note any deviation of the line representing the child's growth from the other percentiles; excessive weight gain should be checked and a falling off in height and weight require investigation. A common presentation is when mother brings a child who appears to eat 'nothing' and whom she thinks is small or light for his age. It is reassuring to both mother and doctor to find the child within the normal range. one reading, however, means little since it is progressive development which is important. If, after 6 months his position on the percentile line is maintained then this is usually sufficient reassurance.

311 This is a common worry in mothers as the tongue is always short at birth and the normal frenulum is more prominent. As the infant grows the tongue lengthens and becomes thin-

149

ner towards the tip and eventually the frenulum is placed well beneath the tip.

Many mothers attribute indistinctness of speech or feeding difficulties to this normal stage of development. True tongue-tie is extremely rare and operation is never indicated until 2 years of age.

The indication for referral is if the child cannot touch the palate or if there is a marked midline depression at the tip and the child cannot lick his upper lip.

312  Anxiety regarding gait is a common presenting problem. Many parents are not aware or have not been told that variations may occur and expect their child to have the legs and gait of an adult as soon as they can walk. It is when the child is 2 years old and over when mother usually brings him stating he is 'knock-kneed' or 'tripping-up all the time'.

Your management depends upon which of the three categories the child falls:

(a)  physiological normal limits.
(b)  within physiological limits but requiring specific measures such as alteration of shoes.
(c)  abnormal and requiring specialist referral.

Diagnosis as usual depends on a good history and full examination.

One aspect of history particularly important is namely achievement of milestones.

Respect for the child during the examination is extremely important. Some degree of undress is important but it should take place gradually and being aware of the child's innate modesty. Observe the child walking with his shoes on. If he does not go to the consulting room door and back on his own he will usually do so with his mother. The procedure is repeated after removal of progressive layers of clothing. Do not fail to examine the shoes.

Individual management of any discovered problem is obviously dependent on the physical diagnosis and also the degree of anxiety of the parents. Where a high level of anxiety exists or the diagnosis is in doubt then therapeutic referral is indicated.

313  The general practitioner with the opportunities

he has to observe interpersonal relationships and social conditions is ideally suited to assess any sexual behaviour which is brought to his attention. He may decide this is normal considering the child's age and family background and so relieve maternal anxiety.

Some adoptive parents have been known to become alarmed when they notice masturbation particularly in girls and a common fear is that they have inherited 'bad blood'. On the other hand if such activity interfered with school or play activities then this would be considered abnormal and the child/family inter-relationship would need to be more closely assessed. There may be merely a family management problem or an early stage of psychosis. Persisting or compulsive behaviour such as exhibitionism, bestiality or sexual assault are rare activities which require referral.

314    The greatest single problem is establishing a sensitive and meaningful doctor/patient relationship. Many adults, including doctors look upon adolescents as sulky potential vandals or dull, uncommunicative children. This is mainly due to insufficient respect being paid to patients of all ages. The adolescent identifies the GP as being 'in league' with his parents and will not respect the confidentiality of his consultation. He might perhaps also think that the doctor's attitude will be a biased one and similar to that of his parents because of their longer standing relationship and similarity of ages.

Although often putting on a worldly face most of these youngsters are very insecure and easily disturbed by an off-hand consultation. Myth and folk-lore loom large in teenage concepts of health care. Lack of family planning leads to unwanted pregnancies and other young one-parent families, teenage marriages, or other long term psychological sequelae. Excessive smoking and drinking cause other health problems and unresolved emotional problems lead to parasuicide and mental breakdown.

315    A 'wet dream' or nocturnal emission is a spontaneous ejaculation occurring during sleep. According to Kinsey 83% of males experience these sometime during their lifetime.

They tend to occur once or twice per month during adolescence. The frequency decreases when sexual intercourse occurs on a regular basis or if masturbation takes place.

They result from spontaneous brain activity during REM sleep, when penile erection takes place. Nocturnal erection phases last on average 25 minutes and occur about every 85 minutes. The proportion of erection time decreases with age.

It is therefore essential to explain to the mother that this is a perfectly normal occurrence in a growing male.

316 (a) Weight—this is an opportunity to discuss weight reduction if necessary and guidance regarding animal fat intake.

(b) Blood pressure—a normal blood pressure, i.e. diastolic level below 95 mmHg would be reassuring. If elevated then the patient needs to return for a follow-up check. It is essential to follow these patients up and defaulters may need to be visited to ensure supervision.

(c) Urine—check random sample for albumin and glucose.

(d) Blood for haemoglobin and serum lipids—fasted specimen required.

(e) Cervical cytology—this should be repeated at annual intervals until two negative results are obtained and then 3-yearly thereafter until the age of 65 years.

(f) Breast examination should be performed and the patient shown how to carry this out herself.

(g) General habits should be raised particularly exercise, smoking and alcohol.

(h) Although the clinic is for 'well-women' many of the attenders come with problems and anxieties they felt were not real illnesses, e.g. anxieties over cancer of the cervix or hypertension. This is equally common if a nurse runs the session. It is therefore important to give these ladies an opportunity to raise any worries and discuss them with due respect.

317 (a) To define their geriatric workload and mobilize available resources such as commun-

ity nursing, flexible appointments systems, surgery access to meet this need.

(b) To compile an at-risk register and discuss this with other members of the practice team, e.g. health visitor.

(c) To educate patients and their relatives in the changing physiology and needs of the elderly.

(d) To maximize each patient's physical and mental ability and by use of the practice team and other agencies such as social services, to maintain the patient in his home environment for as long as possible.

(e) To prevent avoidable problems such as drug overdose and abuse and also such conditions as hypothermia.

318 (a) Isolation—this can be physical, psychological or social. The present family structure makes it increasingly difficult for children to allocate space in their house for elderly parents. In addition it is common for both adults to work so leaving little possibility for supervision during the day. The elderly as a group also tend to make new friends less readily and this inflexibility of attitude contributes to the loneliness. Suicide is common particularly in older men.

(b) Bereavement—because of the very nature of their age then their friends eventually die and grief reactions are frequent.

(c) Retirement—this involves a change in role, e.g. a bank manager, teacher or doctor suddenly feels society no longer needs him. Activities become limited and difficult. They have no role and a diminished income.

(d) Illness—multiple pathology is common in this age group. Many are so stoical as not to mention symptoms or problems until health is permanently affected. The problem is worst in the poorer social classes and less well educated. Diminishing intelligence contributes to the problems and is compounded by a deteriorating personality. Usually the worst aspects of a character profile are magnified.

(e) Intolerance of medication. Here the elderly are similar to young children. Excessive reactions and frequent side effects are com-

monplace. Great caution must be exerted
and side effects looked for at an early stage.
Simplicity of dosage is a maxim.
(f) Limited resources hamper attempts to control fully all the problems mentioned above
and crises develop and in many cases even
crises cannot be dealt with immediately.

319 In a 'typical' practice population of 2400 there
will be 15% over the age of 65, i.e. 360. Of these
125 will be men and 235 women. Over 75 years
then women outnumber men by 3 to 1. It is in
the over 75s that the problems of the elderly
significantly increase.

This is the philosophy behind the aspirations
to increase the total number of general practitioners and decrease the list size to 1600–1700
per GP.

In the 65–70 year age group 12% are unable
to live at home without assistance. This increases to 80% in the 80–85 years age group.

In the practice population of over 65 years of
age 94% live at home looked after by general
practitioners. In the average practice 40% of
consultations are for patients over 65 years.

The above statistics are nationwide averages.
There is considerable weighting in retirement
areas such as seaside resorts and an increase in
the usage of primary care facilities where there
is a bias towards the lower social classes.

320 (a) Organization of the correct place for the
death to take place. This depends on facilities and relatives' feelings but principally
the wishes of the patient.
(b) Control of pain. About 40% of terminally ill
patients experience pain. Analgesia must
be early and adequate to prevent breakdown of confidence.
(c) Control of side effects of analgesics and
other symptoms. These can be as dis-
concerting as the pain, e.g. constipation,
mental confusion, vomiting, nausea. In addition there may be loss of bowel and
bladder control and severe bed-sores. According to one survey 60% of dying
patients have severe physical restrictions
for their last 3 months of life and 20% are
confined to bed.

154

(d) Isolation—patients may be physically alone but often it is a lack of communication with relatives and medical personnel. Discussion of the future is carefully avoided because of upset to both parties.

(e) Support for the relatives. This needs to be both physical and emotional. Discussion must be comprehensive and adequate time allowed.

(f) There are several normal stages which are usually progressed through. These should first of all be understood so that the general practitioner can help the patient: denial; anger; bargaining; depression; acceptance.

(g) The doctor has usually an intimate relationship with the terminally ill either because of the nature of the illness or because of the length of time they have known and trusted each other. Not all of us are equally well equipped to deal with the death of patients we have known well and of whom we have become fond.

321 There are of course no hard and fast rules and it is usually approached by making an 'offer'. An example would be to ask 'Is there anything you wish to ask me?' This may be accepted or rejected. If the latter is the case then it may be because the patient suspects the diagnosis and desires not to face it or because he would rather not know. If the patient genuinely wishes to know then you have no right to deny him the knowledge. It is a difficult area for both doctor and patient to approach and discuss. Great use can be made of non-verbal communication. Compassion can be expressed by eye contact, body gestures, holding the patient's hand or putting an arm around him. Honesty is a vital ingredient but most patients like an escape clause and this is a useful thing to offer. Remember not all patients succumb as quickly as their doctors' believe. Explanations should be couched in language the patient understands, bearing in mind age, sex, social class and your relationship with the person. Some consultations will be very lengthy, do not attempt to rush them.

The main element to be remembered is to be responsive to the patient's feelings and mood. Do not be morose if the patient is optimistic and humorous; do not be flippant if the patient is tearful. Whilst there is sadness in terminal illness the doctor–patient bond is never potentially greater.

322 (a) An experienced social worker will assess the patient in his home with his family or will see him in the department.
(b) Provision of bath attendant.
(c) Organization of the home help service.
(d) Provision of meals on wheels.
(e) An occupational therapist will assess the patient at home and recommend provision of aids. These will be fitted by the local authority under the supervision of the occupational therapist.
(f) They will arrange part III accommodation when available and in conjunction with the general practitioner assess the urgency for this. They can organise holiday relief on such accommodation for relatives of the elderly who cope at home with patients most of the time.
(g) Organization of day care facilities when available and where necessary.

# THE PRACTICE AND PRACTICE ORGANIZATION

323 *Advantages:* regular predictable workload with fewer people kept waiting and, therefore, requiring smaller waiting areas. The general noise and anxiety levels are reduced. Usually there is a feeling of having adequate time allocated to each patient as this can be predetermined. The patient can make an appointment in advance with the doctor of their choice, therefore, predicting a mutually suitable time.

*Disadvantages:* inflexibility occurs and prevents acute problems being seen early and creates anxiety in many patients. This can provoke patient–receptionist battles. The ability to plan ahead operates against three major groups in the community:

(a) children who can become ill rapidly,
(b) the elderly,

(c) the less intelligent who do not understand an appointment system.

Gaps in valuable surgery time may occur as a result of poor time-keeping, forgetful patients and last minute cancellations.

324 (a) Good clinical records. The average general practitioner has a list size of a little under 2400 patients and each patient has a medical record card which is updated with each consultation. This information can be reviewed but this is impossible without cross-indexing. It is not possible otherwise to retrieve information about special diseases in particular age groups. The additional indices necessary are:

(b) An age/sex register—the practice population broken down by age and sex.

(c) A disease register or population index.

325 (a) The details on the front should contain the name, address and date of birth of the patient. Additionally there should be the NHS number, the name of the doctor with whom registered and the date of registration. Extra details of help would be patient's telephone number, occupation and any serious problems, e.g. diabetes, hypertension, allergy etc. Coded tags for the latter problem would be helpful.

(b) A summary record card of significant events.

(c) A prescription record of drugs issued.

(d) Continuation record cards of individual consultations in date order and treasury tagged for convenience.

(e) Significant hospital letters in date order, fastened together.

(f) Investigation results of importance in date order and fastened together.

(g) Perhaps most important of all the writing should be legible and the entries brief but comprehensive.

326 (a) When minor self-limiting illness is presented and simple health education given then very brief details need to be entered perhaps only one or two words.

157

(b) In the case of less serious illness when treatment is prescribed then a two line entry is necessary, namely diagnosis and management.

(c) Entries appertaining to serious illness or chronic disease management require more comprehensive recording. Here we use what has become known as the SOAP convention:

S—for subjective—the patient's stated symptoms or problem.

O—for objective—your findings on examination, both physical and laboratory.

A—assessment—your diagnosis or problem assessment.

P—plan—immediate and long term management in terms of prescription, observations and referral if indicated.

It is useful to include significant diagnoses in (b) and (c) inside a 'box' □ or in a different colour ink.

327 The age/sex register is the practice population sorted as to age and sex. Each section is composed of either males or females with the same year of birth. Commonly it is a card-index system where each patient is represented by an individual card and this contains their date of birth. These cards are sorted in date order with those patients born in January at the front of the section and subsequently through to December 31st.

Some practices are now keeping patients' age/sex characteristics on computer which not only saves space, but also speeds up retrieval of information.

328 There are two main procedures.

(a) Persuade the Family Practitioner Committee to compile the card index system. The ability of any FPC to do this will depend on their available time and local policy. In most cases they will do this but the waiting list for this facility may be prohibitive. GPs working in Scotland can request such a complete register on 'floppy disc' which will be compatible with most computers.

(b) Ancillary staff may compile a register. This means laboriously sorting and noting all patients' records and storing the data either on individual cards or on computer discs. In some cases, extra help can be acquired via the local authority supported personnel, e.g. work experience projects. Many local DHSS offices are helpful in this respect.

329   In any research project it is essential to define the population to be studied and in most cases extract controls which are of a similar age and of the same sex. Unless such a register is available, this is an impossible task.

330   Almost 30% of all prescriptions are written for drugs acting on the nervous system. Tranquillizers, and here Valium heads the list, account for 27% of these. Of prescriptions in this group 24% are for analgesics while 23% are for hypnotics and 11% for antidepressants.

Antibiotics are the next largest group comprising 15% of overall prescribing with penicillins 47% of this group and tetracyclines 26%.

Cardiovascular drugs form 11% of the total with diuretics 37% of this group, cardiac preparations 23% and antihypertensives 20%.

331   (a) It must be cheap, simple and easy to administer.
(b) The record should show what drugs were last prescribed and when and what quantity.
(c) There should be an inbuilt capacity to check that the patient is taking the drug in the quantity prescribed.
(d) There should be feedback to the doctor of what drugs he is prescribing and in what quantities.
(e) The patient should understand the workings of the system and be able to obtain the prescription requested within a reasonable period of time (usually 24 hours).
(f) There should be an emergency back-up capability, because of failure of either patient to remember or system to comply, whereby the patient can obtain a necessary drug quickly.

332 (a) Placing a suggestion box encourages feedback of problems. Some suggestions may be frivolous but all are worth serious consideration.
   (b) Compile a news sheet which lists the services available and the characteristics of the practice and place these in the waiting room. If possible enrol a patient as the editor and encourage contributions from other patients for inclusion.
   (c) Encourage the formation of a patient participation group which will consist mainly of patients but with staff and doctor representation. Preferably a patient should be chairman. This will act as an avenue for complaints but also objective advice will be forthcoming about practice policy. Other activities may include:

   (i) transport service for the rural areas.
   (ii) prescription delivery for the elderly or isolated.
   (iii) hospital visiting service.
   (iv) night sitting service.
   (v) volunteers to help with visiting service for elderly and housebound.

   (d) Organization of self-care groups, e.g. diabetics, smokers, hypertensives, slimmers etc.

333 All reactions to recently introduced drugs, vaccines, surgical materials, IUCDs, absorbable sutures and even contact lenses must be reported to the Committee on Safety of Medicines. The report is made on a 'yellow card' which is reply-paid. It is particularly important in the case of recently introduced drugs and these are identified in the British National Formulary by a black triangle.

   In addition all suspected drug interactions should be reported. The supply of yellow cards is direct from the Committee on Safety of Medicines and these are sent by return after a notification. Feedback as to how common the problem is which you have identified is available from the Committee by ticking a box on the 'yellow form'.

334 This group includes such medicines as pethidine, morphine, amphetamines, methaqualone etc.

The prescriber must do the following.

(a) Write in ink or some other indelible substance and it must be signed and dated by him.
(b) The name and address of the patient should be in the prescriber's own handwriting.
(c) The name and address of the prescriber must be present on the prescription.
(d) The dose to be taken must be in the prescriber's handwriting, as must the form of the drug, e.g. tablet or syrup. If there is more than one strength then this must always appear. The prescription must also specify either the total quantity of the drug to be supplied or the total number of dosage units in both words and figures.

335  (a) She is especially able to assess the nursing needs of a patient in the home situation and report back to the other primary care team members.
(b) She is able to record clinical information and together with other members of the primary care team coordinate and supervise a nursing management plan.
(c) With adequate training and supervision she can perform more skilled diagnostic procedures such as ECG recording and venepuncture.
(d) Undertake treatment including first-aid.
(e) Perform general nursing care and supervise the work of other members of the team, e.g. bath attendant, SENs etc.
(f) With the special role she has in the community she can help reinforce health education and general advice given by the doctor or health visitor and help present a 'united front' from the point of view of preventive care.
(g) She is a powerful support to relatives looking after sick patients.

336  There are four main elements.

(a) The family practitioners are coordinated by the local medical committee.
(b) The pharmaceutical services are organized by the Area Chemists Contractors Committee which are responsible to the FPC.

(c) Ophthalmic services—organized by the Local Optical Committee.

(d) Dental services—supervised by the local dental committee.

337 (a) To organize the contractual duty of general practitioners to provide general medical services in the area.

(b) To select general practitioners and to appoint them after consideration. Also to control the number present in the area under supervision.

(c) To pay general practitioners.

(d) To display lists of general practitioners so that members of the public are able to see their range of choice.

(e) To investigate complaints against general practitioners in respect of terms of service.

(f) To record patient movement between practitioners in the area and between areas.

(g) To allocate patients to individual doctors' lists.

(h) To pass on items of information regarding terms of service and aspects of remuneration.

338 (a) To render to his patients all proper and necessary treatments and advice which is within the competence, experience and limitations of any general practitioner.

(b) To prescribe adequate, proper and sufficient drugs, dressings and appliances as may be necessary.

(c) To arrange further treatment by hospital, community physician or other practitioner services if required.

(d) To give immediate emergency treatment if a patient's own doctor is not available.

(e) To attend and treat all patients on his list at the places agreed with the Family Practitioner Committee. He may defer treatment if there is no detriment to the patient but he is responsible for a deputy acting on his behalf.

(f) To provide adequate practice premises with waiting room facilities.

(g) To visit and treat a patient at home.

(h) To issue all certificates as required by law.

(i) To keep proper records, on correct forms of all illnesses and treatments.

(j) To provide clinical information to the Regional Medical Officer and assist him in his duties.

(k) To ensure that if absent his terms of service will be covered by a deputy for whom he is responsible.

339 (a) They may merely admonish the doctor and close the case.

(b) They may place the doctor on probation by postponing judgement for a defined period. He will be allowed to practice unrestricted during the interim period.

(c) They may order that the doctor's registration shall be subject to his compliance, for a period not exceeding 3 years, with specified conditions of service.

(d) They may direct that the doctor's registration shall be suspended for a period not exceeding 12 months.

(e) They may direct erasure.

340 (a) Request independent published audience. It is very difficult to interpret clinical tests quickly. Ask for reviewed articles such as published in *Prescribers Journal*, or *Drug and Therapeutics Bulletin*, or leaders in the *BMJ*. Promotion brochures are often biased with simplified histograms and incomplete extracts.

(b) Evaluate the evidence. Important improvements should be substantiated by independent review articles and clinical trials of adequate size in countries which have a similar population structure, preferably the UK. Before changing, the advantages must be significant.

(c) If the new drug costs more then it should be significantly better. If the effect is similar then choose the cheapest. Many manufacturers change the product slightly but claim an improvement where the product licence is running out. This extends the patent and maintains a share in the market.

A drug representative from a reputable company has access to enormous amounts of useful information about products. This knowledge is there for the asking.

# 4

# Reading List

The most important learning tool which any student of whatever age has at his disposal is the material with which he is working at the time. In the case of medical students this is of course his patient population. An enormous amount about any disease process or aspects of human behaviour can be learnt from simply talking and listening to patients in a disciplined manner. Whatever problem the patient has then read around the subject later using the actual patient's problems as knowledge 'hatpegs'.

In addition I have found the following magazines extremely useful and they are of course absolutely up to date unlike the more conventional texts.

*The British Medical Journal*
*Update*
*Medicine*
*The Prescribers Journal*
*Drug and Therapeutics Bulletin*
*The Practitioner.*

I make no apologies for missing out more prestigious journals as I find it sufficiently difficult to keep up to date with those mentioned above and it simply is not possible to read them all.

In compiling the questions I have referred to my favourite standard works and they are listed under Bibliography. I cannot recommend them too highly especially those dedicated to general practice. If you have time remaining READ THEM. After you have read them GOOD LUCK.

# 5
# Bibliography

*Drug and Therapeutics Bulletin*
*Essential Ophthalmology.* Chawla, H. B. (Churchill Livingstone, Edinburgh, 1981)
*General Ophthalmology.* Vaughan, D. and Asbury, T. (Lange Medical Publications, California, 1980)
*Language and Communication in General Practice.* Ed. Tanner, B. A. (Hodder and Stoughton, London, 1977)
*The Normal Child, Some Problems of the Early Years and their Treatment.* Illingworth, R. S. (Churchill Livingstone, Edinburgh, 1979)
*The Oxford Textbook of Medicine.* Eds. Weatherall, D. J., Ledingham, J. G. G. and Warrel, D. A. (Oxford University Press, 1983)
*Practice—A Handbook of Primary Medical Care.* Eds. Cormack, J. J. C., Marinker, M. L. and Morrell, D. C. (Kluwer-Harrop Handbooks, London, 1982)
*The Practitioner*
*The Prescribers Journal*
*Problems of Childhood.* (British Medical Journal, London, 1976)
*The Journal of the Royal College of General Practitioners*
*The Scientific Foundations of Family Medicine.* Eds. Fry, J., Gambrill E. and Smith, R. (William Heinemann Medical Books Ltd, London, 1978)
*Towards Earlier Diagnosis in Primary Care.* Hodgkin, K. (Churchill Livingstone, Edinburgh, 1978)
*Treatment—A Handbook of Drug Therapy.* Eds. Drury, V. W. M., Wade, O. L., Beely, L., and Alesbury, P. (Kluwer Publishing Ltd. London)
*Update*